Safer Prescribing

Safer Prescribing
a guide to some problems in the use of drugs

Linda Beeley
MA, FRCP
Drug and Therapeutics Unit
Queen Elizabeth Hospital
Birmingham

FIFTH EDITION

OXFORD

Blackwell Scientific Publications

LONDON EDINBURGH BOSTON

MELBOURNE PARIS BERLIN VIENNA

© 1976, 1979, 1983, 1987, 1992 by
Blackwell Scientific Publications
Editorial Offices:
Osney Mead, Oxford OX2 0EL
25 John Street, London WC1N 2BL
23 Ainslie Place, Edinburgh EH3 6AJ
3 Cambridge Center, Cambridge
 Massachusetts 02142, USA
54 University Street, Carlton
 Victoria 3053, Australia

Other Editorial Offices:
Librairie Arnette SA
2, rue Casimir-Delavigne
75006 Paris
France

Blackwell Wissenschafts-Verlag
Meinekestrasse 4
D-1000 Berlin 15
Germany

Blackwell MZV
Feldgasse 13
A-1238 Wien
Austria

First published 1976
Reprinted 1977, 1978
Second edition 1979
Reprinted 1981
German edition 1981
Spanish edition 1981
French edition 1982
Dutch edition 1982
Third edition 1983
Reprinted 1984, 1985
Fourth edition 1987
Reprinted 1988, 1990
German edition 1989
Fifth edition 1992

Set by Excel Typesetters, Hong Kong
Printed and bound in Great Britain at
The Alden Press, Oxford

DISTRIBUTORS

Marston Book Services Ltd
PO Box 87
Oxford OX2 0DT
(*Orders*: Tel. 0865 791155
 Fax: 0865 791927
 Telex: 837515)

USA
Blackwell Scientific Publications,
Inc.
3 Cambridge Center
Cambridge, MA 02142
(*Orders*: Tel: 800 759-6102)

Canada
Times Mirror Professional
Publishing, Ltd.
5240 Finch Avenue East
Scarborough, Ontario M1S 5A2
(*Orders*: Tel: 416 298-1588)

Australia
Blackwell Scientific Publications
(Australia) Pty Ltd
54 University Street
Carlton, Victoria 3053
(*Orders*: Tel: 03 347-0300)

British Library
Cataloguing in Publication Data

Beeley, Linda
 Safer prescribing.—5th ed
 I. Title
 615.704

 ISBN 0-632-03292-8

Contents

Preface to fifth edition

The book has been extensively revised to include information about new drugs and new information about older drugs.

I should like to thank Margaret Rea for her help in preparing this edition.

As before, I will supply references to specific points on request.

Linda Beeley

Preface to first edition

My intention in this booklet is to provide an easy reference source of information for some of the factors which can lead to problems in drug prescribing.

The tables are not comprehensive, but should contain most of the clinically important information.

References are not given, but I will supply them on specific points on request.

Linda Beeley

List of abbreviations

ACE	angiotensin-converting enzyme
ACTH	adrenocorticotrophic hormone
AV	atrioventricular
CNS	central nervous sytem
GFR	glomerular filtration rate
G6PD	glucose-6-phosphate dehydrogenase
IV	intravenous
MAOIs	monoamine oxidase inhibitors
NSAIDs	non-steroidal anti-inflammatory drugs

Drug interactions

Drug interactions are of two kinds:

1 Pharmacodynamic interactions occur between drugs which compete for the same receptor site or act on the same physiological system. They can also occur indirectly when a drug-induced disease or change in fluid or electrolyte balance alters the response to another drug.

2 Pharmacokinetic interactions occur when one drug alters the absorption, distribution or elimination of another drug such that the amount which reaches the site of action is increased or decreased. It is generally true that pharmacodynamic interactions demonstrated with one drug should be anticipated with related drugs. Pharmacokinetic interactions, on the other hand, cannot be extrapolated to combinations of pharmacologically related drugs unless the pharmacokinetics are known to be similar.

From the therapeutic point of view the result of a drug interaction can be harmful, unimportant or useful. The following tables list those interactions that have been shown to be or are potentially harmful in humans during normal clinical use of the drugs concerned. They are not intended to be comprehensive lists of all possible interactions, and therapeutically useful interactions are not included. In most of the tables the drug whose action is affected is listed in column 1 and drugs are arranged by body system. Column 2 lists the drugs that interact with the primary drug, and column 3 states the mechanism and result of the interaction.

Because only the drug affected appears in column 1, when using the tables to check whether any interaction is likely to occur between drugs prescribed for a patient each drug must be looked for in column 1 and the presence of the others sought in column 2.

The table of drug interactions with alcohol differs from the others as it contains all drug–alcohol interactions, regardless of whether it is the effect of the drug or the effect of alcohol which changes.

ALIMENTARY SYSTEM

DRUGS AFFECTED	DRUGS WHICH INTERACT	RESULT OF INTERACTION
Carbenoxolone	Amiloride Spironolactone	Inhibition of ulcer healing.

DRUGS AFFECTED	DRUGS WHICH INTERACT	RESULT OF INTERACTION
Cimetidine	Rifampicin	Increased cimetidine metabolism and lower plasma concentration.
Metoclopramide Domperidone Cisapride	Anticholinergic drugs, e.g. propantheline benzhexol Opioid analgesics	Antagonize the effect on gastrointestinal motility.

CARDIOVASCULAR SYSTEM

Cardiac glycosides, e.g. digoxin digitoxin	Diuretics: thiazides loop diuretics Carbenoxolone Amphotericin	Toxicity increased by hypokalaemia.
	Verapamil	Increased bradycardia and AV block.
	Cholestyramine Colestipol	Reduced absorption. Give at least 3 h apart.
	Quinidine Quinine Amiodarone Propafenone	Increased plasma concentration of digoxin and risk of toxicity. Dose of digoxin should be halved.
	Diltiazem Nicardipine Spironolactone Verapamil Chloroquine	Have been reported to increase the plasma concentration of digoxin.
	Erythromycin	Increased effect of digoxin.

DRUGS AFFECTED	DRUGS WHICH INTERACT	RESULT OF INTERACTION
	Antacids	Have been shown to reduce the absorption of digoxin. Clinical importance probably small.
	NSAIDs	May increase plasma concentration by reducing GFR.
	Calcium salts	Large IV doses can precipitate arrhythmias.
	Phenobarbitone Phenytoin Rifampicin Aminoglutethimide	Reduced effect of digitoxin due to increased metabolism.

Diuretics

DRUGS AFFECTED	DRUGS WHICH INTERACT	RESULT OF INTERACTION
Thiazides Frusemide Bumetanide Ethacrynic acid Piretanide Xipamide	Acetazolamide Indapamide Corticosteroids, ACTH Carbenoxolone	Increased urinary potassium loss and risk of hypokalaemia.
	NSAIDS, e.g. indomethacin piroxicam Carbenoxolone Oestrogens Corticosteroids, ACTH	Diuretic effect antagonized by fluid retention.
Frusemide	Metolazone	Profound diuresis and electrolyte disturbance can occur.

DRUGS AFFECTED	DRUGS WHICH INTERACT	RESULT OF INTERACTION
Thiazides	Cholestyramine	Reduced absorption. Give at least 2 h apart.
Amiloride Spironolactone Triamterene	Potassium supplements ACE inhibitors Cyclosporin Indomethacin and possibly other NSAIDs	Increased risk of hyperkalaemia, especially if renal function is impaired.
Spironolactone	Aspirin Indomethacin	Inhibition of natriuretic effect—mechanism unknown.
Potassium-sparing diuretic + thiazide combined preparations, e.g. Moduretic	Chlorpropamide	Increased risk of hyponatraemia.

Antiarrhythmic drugs

	Concurrent use of two or more	Increased risk of myocardial depression, hypotension, heart failure, conduction defects, ventricular arrhythmias.
	Beta-adrenoceptor antagonists	Increased risk of myocardial depression, hypotension, heart failure, conduction defects, asystole.

DRUGS AFFECTED	DRUGS WHICH INTERACT	RESULT OF INTERACTION
Disopyramide Flecainide Procainamide Quinidine	Amiodarone	Increased risk of ventricular arrhythmias. Increased plasma concentration of procainamide, quinidine and flecainide.
Amiodarone	Diltiazem Verapamil	Increased risk of bradycardia, AV block and myocardial depression.
Amiodarone Disopyramide Flecainide Quinidine	Diuretics: thiazides loop diuretics Carbenoxolone	Increased risk of ventricular arrhythmias in the presence of hypokalaemia.
Lignocaine Mexiletine Tocainide	Diuretics: thiazides loop diuretics	Less effective in the presence of hypokalaemia.
Lignocaine	Cimetidine Propranolol	Reduced clearance of lignocaine and increased risk of toxicity.
Mexiletine	Atropine Opioid analgesics	Delayed absorption. Can be overcome by giving a larger (oral) loading dose of mexiletine.
	Metoclopramide	Increased rate of absorption of mexiletine.
	Rifampicin Phenytoin	Increased metabolism and lower plasma concentration of mexiletine.

DRUGS AFFECTED	DRUGS WHICH INTERACT	RESULT OF INTERACTION
Mexiletine Quinidine Flecainide	Antacids Acetazolamide	Reduced excretion in alkaline urine may occasionally increase plasma concentrations. Toxicity could occur.
Flecainide Procainamide Quinidine Amiodarone Propafenone	Cimetidine	Increased plasma concentration.
Quinidine	Verapamil	Increased plasma concentration of quinidine. Extreme hypotension can occur.
	Phenobarbitone Phenytoin Primidone Rifampicin	Increased metabolism and lower plasma concentration of quinidine.
Propafenone	Quinidine	Increased plasma concentration.
	Rifampicin	Reduced plasma concentration.
Verapamil	Rifampicin	Increased metabolism and lower plasma concentration.
Disopyramide	Anticholinergic drugs, e.g. antidepressants antiparkinsonism drugs propantheline	Increased anticholinergic side-effects—dry mouth, urine retention, etc.

DRUGS AFFECTED	DRUGS WHICH INTERACT	RESULT OF INTERACTION
	Rifampicin Phenobarbitone Primidone Phenytoin	Increased metabolism and reduced plasma concentration.
	Erythromycin	Increased plasma concentration and risk of toxicity.

Beta-adrenoceptor antagonists

All (see also Antihypertensive drugs)	Digoxin	Increased AV block and bradycardia.

	Sympathomimetic amines, e.g.
	   adrenaline
	   noradrenaline
	   phenylpropanol-
	      amine
	   phenylephrine
	   (present in
	      proprietary
	      common cold
	      remedies)
		Severe hypertension can occur.

	Verapamil	Increased risk of myocardial depression, hypotension, bradycardia, asystole.
	Nifedipine	Severe hypotension and heart failure can occur occasionally.
	Diltiazem	Increased risk of bradycardia and AV block.

DRUGS AFFECTED	DRUGS WHICH INTERACT	RESULT OF INTERACTION
	Amiodarone	Increased risk of bradycardia and AV block.
	Ergotamine	Increased risk of peripheral vasoconstriction.
Propranolol	Cimetidine	Reduced clearance, increased plasma concentration and increased risk of bradycardia.
	Thyroxine	Increased metabolism, and lower plasma concentration of propranolol. Higher doses may be needed.
	Rifampicin	Increased metabolism and lower plasma concentration.
	Fluvoxamine	Increased plasma concentration.
	Reserpine	Increased bradycardia.
	Digoxin	Increased bradycardia and AV block.
Sotalol	Diuretics: thiazides loop diuretics	Increased risk of ventricular arrhythmias in the presence of hypokalaemia.

DRUGS AFFECTED	DRUGS WHICH INTERACT	RESULT OF INTERACTION
Antihypertensive drugs		
All	NSAIDs, e.g. indomethacin piroxicam Carbenoxolone Corticosteroids, ACTH Oral contraceptives	Hypotensive effect antagonized by drugs causing fluid retention or hypertension.
	Alcohol Sedatives and hypnotics Phenothiazines Antidepressants (but see below) Levodopa Fenfluramine Nitrates Calcium-channel blockers Baclofen Peripheral vasodilators Diuretics	Potentiation. These drugs all produce hypotension as a side effect.
Bethanidine Debrisoquine Guanethidine	Tricyclic antidepressants Indirect sympathomimetic amines, e.g. amphetamines phenylpropanol-amine (present in proprietary common cold remedies) Mazindol Pizotifen	Antagonism. Neuronal uptake to site of action is prevented.

DRUGS AFFECTED	DRUGS WHICH INTERACT	RESULT OF INTERACTION
Clonidine	Tricyclic antidepressants	Antagonism. Probably a central effect. Also may potentiate withdrawal hypertension.
	Beta-adrenoceptor antagonists	Can potentiate withdrawal hypertension. When changing from clonidine to a beta-blocker several days should be left between stopping clonidine and starting the beta-blocker.
Labetalol	Cimetidine	Reduced clearance and increased plasma concentration.
Prazosin Terazosin Doxazosin	Beta-adrenoceptor antagonists Diuretics	Increased postural hypotensive effect of initial dose.
ACE inhibitors	Potassium salts Potassium-sparing diuretics Indomethacin and possibly other NSAIDs Cyclosporin	Increased risk of hyperkalaemia.
	Probenecid	Reduced excretion of captopril.
	Diuretics	Potentiation and risk of extreme hypotension.

DRUGS AFFECTED	DRUGS WHICH INTERACT	RESULT OF INTERACTION
	NSAIDs	Increased risk of renal failure.
Indapamide	Diuretics: thiazides loop diuretics Carbenoxolone	Increased risk of hypokalaemia.

Vasodilators
(for verapamil see Antiarrhythmics)

DRUGS AFFECTED	DRUGS WHICH INTERACT	RESULT OF INTERACTION
Diltiazem Nicardipine Nifedipine Felodipine	Cimetidine	Increased plasma concentrations due to inhibition of metabolism.
Nifedipine Nicardipine Isradipine Felodipine	Carbamazepine	Reduced plasma concentrations.
Glyceryl trinitrate (sublingual)	Anticholinergic drugs, e.g. tricyclic antidepressants phenothiazines disopyramide propantheline	Loss of effect due to failure to dissolve in a dry mouth.

Vasoconstrictors

DRUGS AFFECTED	DRUGS WHICH INTERACT	RESULT OF INTERACTION
Noradrenaline Adrenaline	Tricyclic antidepressants	Potentiation due to inhibition of neuronal uptake. Hypertension, tachycardia, arrhythmias may occur.

DRUGS AFFECTED	DRUGS WHICH INTERACT	RESULT OF INTERACTION
	Guanethidine Reserpine	Potentiation due to increased receptor sensitivity (denervation supersensitivity).
	Beta-adrenoceptor antagonists	Potentiation of hypertensive effect
Metaraminol Phenylephrine	Bethanidine Debrisoquine Guanethidine Reserpine	Potentiation of direct vasoconstrictor effect. Hypertension may occur. N.B. Phenylephrine is present in many proprietary common cold remedies.

Anticoagulants

DRUGS AFFECTED	DRUGS WHICH INTERACT	RESULT OF INTERACTION
Heparin	Aspirin Dipyridamole Sulphinpyrazone	Increased risk of bleeding.
Coumarins: warfarin nicoumalone	Cholestyramine	Cholestyramine interfers with the absorption of warfarin and of vitamin K. Either inhibition or potentiation is possible.
	Aminoglutethimide Barbiturates Carbamazepine Griseofulvin Primidone Rifampicin	Reduced anticoagulant effect due to increased metabolism. Overdose and bleeding may occur when interacting drug is stopped.

DRUGS AFFECTED	DRUGS WHICH INTERACT	RESULT OF INTERACTION
	Rowachol	May reduce anticoagulant effect.
	Alcohol (acute intoxication) Amiodarone Chloramphenicol Cimetidine Ciprofloxacin Disulfiram Enoxacin Erythromycin Fluconazole Fluvoxamine Itraconazole Ketoconazole Metronidazole Miconazole Norfloxacin Omeprazole Paroxetine Propafenone Sulphinpyrazone	Increased effect due to inhibition of coumarin metabolism.
	Phenytoin	Both potentiation and inhibition have been reported.
	Co-trimoxazole and possibly other sulphonamides	Increased effect probably due partly to inhibition of metabolism and partly to displacement from protein binding.
	NSAIDs	All can cause gastric erosions and bleeding, and affect platelet function. Avoid if possible (see also below).

DRUGS AFFECTED	DRUGS WHICH INTERACT	RESULT OF INTERACTION
	Phenylbutazone	Increased effect due to inhibition of metabolism and displacement from protein binding. Serious risk of haemorrhage.
	Azapropazone	Resembles phenylbutazone and potentiation has been reported.
	Mefenamic acid Diflunisal Flurbiprofen Sulindac Piroxicam	Potentiation has been reported.
	Indomethacin Diclofenac Fenbufen Fenoprofen Ibuprofen Ketoprofen Naproxen Tiaprofenic acid Tolmetin	These do not appear to interact directly with warfarin.
	Clofibrate Bezafibrate Gemfibrozil Anabolic steriods, e.g. oxymetholone stanozolol Danazol Tamoxifen	Increased effect. Mechanism not established but evidence suggests an interaction at the receptor site.
	Oral broad-spectrum antibiotics	They are said to potentiate anticoagulants by

DRUGS AFFECTED	DRUGS WHICH INTERACT	RESULT OF INTERACTION
		reducing bacterial synthesis of vitamin K, but significant vitamin K deficiency is very unlikely to occur unless dietary vitamin is also reduced and treatment is continued for many weeks. The risk may be greater with tetracyclines than with other antibiotics.
	Cefamandole Aztreonam	Potentiation due to additive hypopro-thrombinaemic effect.
	Thyroxine	Increased metabolism of vitamin K-dependent clotting factors and increased sensitivity to warfarin. A dose reduction may be necessary after treatment of hypothyroidism.
	Aspirin Dipyridamole	Increased risk of bleeding due to anti-platelet effect. A single dose of aspirin can prolong the bleeding time for up to 5 days, and large doses also have a hypoprothrom-binaemic effect.

DRUGS AFFECTED	DRUGS WHICH INTERACT	RESULT OF INTERACTION
	Oral contraceptives	Reduced effect due to increased synthesis of vitamin K-dependent clotting factors.
	Vitamin K	Reversal of anticoagulant effect due to competitive inhibition. N.B. Present in some enteral feeds.
	Sucralfate	Absorption may be reduced
	Allopurinol Chloral hydrate Dextropro- poxyphene (co- proxamol) Paracetamol (prolonged regular use) Proguanil Nalidixic acid Quinidine Lovastatin Simvastatin Vitamin E (high doses)	Potentiation has been reported but clinical importance not established.

Phenindione

Phenindione does not appear to share all the interactions of coumarins. It can be expected to interact in the same way as the coumarins with the following drugs:

DRUGS AFFECTED	DRUGS WHICH INTERACT	RESULT OF INTERACTION
	Aspirin Anabolic steroids Dipyridamole Clofibrate Bezafibrate Gemfibrozil Danazol Thyrozine Oral broad-spectrum antibiotics Cefamandole Cholestyramine	Potentiation—as for coumarins above.
	Oral contraceptives Preparations containing vitamin K	Inhibition—as for coumarins above.

Lipid-lowering drugs

Lovastatin Pravastatin Simvastatin	Cyclosporin Clofibrate Bezafibrate Gemfibrozil	Increased risk of myopathy.

RESPIRATORY SYSTEM

Theophylline	Cimetidine Ciprofloxacin Diltiazem Disulfiram Enoxacin Erythromycin Interferons Isoniazid Mexiletine Norfloxacin Oral contraceptives Viloxazine	Inhibition of theophylline metabolism, increased plasma concentration and risk of toxicity.

DRUGS AFFECTED	DRUGS WHICH INTERACT	RESULT OF INTERACTION
	Aminoglutethimide Barbiturates Carbamazepine Phenytoin Rifampicin Sulphinpyrazone	Increased metabolism and lower plasma concentration of theophylline. Higher doses may be needed.

Sympathomimetic bronchodilators, e.g.
   salbutamol
   terbutaline
	Beta-adrenoceptor antagonists	Antagonism of bronchodilator effect.

	Corticosteroids Theophylline	Increased risk of hypokalaemia with high doses of sympathomimetics.

ANALGESICS AND DRUGS USED IN ARTHRITIS AND GOUT

Pethidine	Cimetidine	Increased plasma concentration due to inhibition of metabolism.
Methadone	Rifampicin	Increased metabolism and lower plasma concentration of methadone.
Alfentanil	Erythromycin	Increased plasma concentration.
Aspirin	Metoclopramide	Increased rate of absorption and higher plasma concentration, especially when absorption is delayed, as in migraine.

DRUGS AFFECTED	DRUGS WHICH INTERACT	RESULT OF INTERACTION
	Antacids (large doses)	Increased renal excretion of aspirin and lower plasma concentration.
Paracetamol	Metoclopramide	As for aspirin.
	Cholestyramine	Reduced absorption.
Nefopam	MAOIs	Possibility of CNS toxicity.
Diflunisal	Antacids	Absorption is significantly reduced by aluminium hydroxide.
NSAIDs (all)	Diuretics	Increased risk of nephrotoxicity.
Indomethain Ketoprofen Naproxen (and probably other NSAIDs)	Probenecid	Reduced excretion and higher plasma concentrations.
Phenylbutazone	Cholestyramine	Reduced absorption
Penicillamine	Antacids Oral iron Zinc sulphate	Reduced absorption of penicillamine. Give at least 3 h apart.
Probenecid Sulphinpyrazone	Aspirin Pyrazinamide	Inhibition of uricosuric effect. In a dose of less than 2 g daily, aspirin also causes uric acid retention.

DRUGS AFFECTED	DRUGS WHICH INTERACT	RESULT OF INTERACTION

CENTRAL NERVOUS SYSTEM

Hypnotics and sedatives

DRUGS AFFECTED	DRUGS WHICH INTERACT	RESULT OF INTERACTION
All	Alcohol Opioid analgesics Antihistamines Baclofen Phenothiazines Antidepressants	Increased CNS depression.
Alprazolam Chlordiazepoxide Clobazam Diazepam Flurazepam Midazolam Nitrazepam Triazolam	Cimetidine	Increased plasma concentrations due to inhibition of benzodiazepine metabolism.
Diazepam Chlordiazepoxide	Disulfiram	Increased plasma concentrations due to inhibition of benzodiazepine metabolism.
Diazepam	Omeprazole	Increased plasma concentration.
Triazolam Midazolam	Erythromycin	Increased plasma concentrations due to inhibition of metabolism.
Chlormethiazole	Cimetidine	Increased plasma concentration due to inhibition of metabolism.

Antipsychotic drugs and lithium

DRUGS AFFECTED	DRUGS WHICH INTERACT	RESULT OF INTERACTION
Antipsychotic drugs (all)	Metoclopramide Reserpine Tetrabenazine	Increased risk of extrapyramidal side-effects.

DRUGS AFFECTED	DRUGS WHICH INTERACT	RESULT OF INTERACTION
Haloperidol	Carbamazepine Rifampicin	Increased metabolism and lower plasma concentration of haloperidol.
	Fluoxetine	Increased plasma concentration of haloperidol.
Phenothiazines	Anticholinergic drugs, e.g. benzhexol benztropine	Increased anti-cholinergic side-effects—dry mouth, urine retention, constipation. Plasma concentrations may be reduced.
	Tricyclic antidepressants	Increased anti-cholinergic side-effects. Plasma concentrations may be increased.
	Cimetidine	Increased plasma concentration of chlorpromazine, clozapine and possibly others.
Chlorpromazine	Aluminium hydroxide Magnesium trisilicate	Absorption of chlorpromazine may be reduced. Clinical importance unknown.
	Propranolol	Increased plasma concentration.

DRUGS AFFECTED	DRUGS WHICH INTERACT	RESULT OF INTERACTION
Pimozide	Diuretics: loop thiazide Carbenoxolone	Increased risk of arrhythmias in the presence of hypokalaemia.
Lithium	Acetazolamide Theophylline	Increased lithium excretion. Dose of lithium may have to be increased.
	Thiazide diuretics	Reduced excretion of lithium and risk of toxicity.
	Loop diuretics, e.g. frusemide	Safer than thiazides but sodium depletion can cause lithium toxicity.
	Sodium bicarbonate Sodium chloride	Large doses increase lithium excretion and reduce the plasma concentration. Sodium depletion increases lithium toxicity.
	NSAIDs	Reduced excretion of lithium and risk of toxicity.
	Haloperidol Phenothiazines Metoclopramide	Increased risk of extrapyramidal reactions and possibly of neurotoxicity.
	Carbamazepine Phenytoin Methyldopa Diltiazem Verapamil	Neurotoxicity has been reported at therapeutic plasma concentrations of lithium.

DRUGS AFFECTED	DRUGS WHICH INTERACT	RESULT OF INTERACTION
	Tricyclic antidepressants Maprotiline	CNS excitation, hypertension and convulsions.
	Tryptophan	CNS excitation, confusional states, myoclonus.
Fluvoxamine Fluoxetine Paroxetine Sertraline	Lithium MAOIs Tryptophan	Increased risk of CNS toxicity.

Anticonvulsants

All	Antipsychotic drugs Antidepressants	Antagonism—these drugs lower the convulsive threshold.
	Methotrexate Co-trimoxazole Trimethoprim Pyrimethamine Oral contraceptives Sulphasalazine	Potentiation of folate deficiency is a possibility.
Phenytoin	Amiodarone Azapropazone Chloramphenicol Cimetidine Co-trimoxazole Cycloserine Disulfiram Ditiazem Fluconazole Isoniazid Ketoconazole Metronidazole Miconazole Omeprazole Phenylbutazone Sulphaphenazole Sulphinpyrazone Trimethoprim Viloxazine	Potentiation and increased toxicity due to inhibition of phenytoin metabolism.

DRUGS AFFECTED	DRUGS WHICH INTERACT	RESULT OF INTERACTION
	Influenza vaccine	Potentiation of phenytoin has been reported.
	Rifampicin	Increased metabolism and lower plasma concentration of phenytoin.
	Carbamazepine Folic acid Phenobarbitone Vigabatrin	Increased phenytoin metabolism. Clinical importance probably small.
	Aspirin Sodium valproate Tolbutamide	Displace phenytoin from protein binding. Potentiation will usually be transient but total plasma concentration used for monitoring therapy will be low in relation to the free concentration.
	Sucralfate Antacids Cytotoxic drugs	Reduced absorption of phenytoin.
Phenobarbitone Primidone	Phenytoin Sodium valproate	Inhibition of phenobarbitone metabolism. Increased plasma concentration of phenobarbitone and increased sedation.
Carbamazepine	Phenobarbitone Phenytoin	Increased metabolism and lower plasma concentration of

DRUGS AFFECTED	DRUGS WHICH INTERACT	RESULT OF INTERACTION
		carbamazepine. Clinical importance probably small.
	Cimetidine Danazol Dextropropoxyphene (co-proxamol) Diltiazem Erythromycin Fluoxetine Isoniazid Sodium valproate Verapamil Viloxazine	Increased plasma concentration and risk of toxicity due to inhibition of carbamazepine metabolism.
Ethosuximide	Carbamazepine	Increased metabolism and lower plasma concentration of ethosuximide.
	Isoniazid Sodium valproate	Inhibition of metabolism and increased plasma concentration of ethosuximide.
Sodium valproate	Carbamazepine Phenytoin Phenobarbitone Primidone	Increased metabolism. Plasma concentration may fall. Clinical importance probably small. Extreme lethargy, stupor and coma have been reported when sodium valproate was given to patients on other anticonvulsants.

DRUGS AFFECTED	DRUGS WHICH INTERACT	RESULT OF INTERACTION
	Aspirin	Risk of toxicity.
Clonazepam	Carbamazepine Phenytoin Phenobarbitone	Increased metabolism and lower plasma concentration.

Drugs used in parkinsonism

DRUGS AFFECTED	DRUGS WHICH INTERACT	RESULT OF INTERACTION
Anticholinergic drugs, e.g. benzhexol orphenadrine	Tricyclic anti-depressants Phenothiazines Monoamine oxidase inhibitors Antihistamines Disopyramide	Increased anticholinergic side-effects—dry mouth, blurred vision, urinary retention, constipation.
	Tricyclic anti-depressants Monoamine oxidase inhibitors Amantadine	Excitement, confusion and hallucinations—additive central anticholinergic effects.
Levodopa	Antipsychotic drugs, e.g. haloperidol phenothiazines Tetrabenazine Reserpine Methyldopa	Antagonism. These drugs have extrapyramidal side-effects.
	Benzodiazepines	Deterioration has been reported in patients on levodopa who were given diazepam, chlordiazepoxide or lorazepam.
	Metoclopramide	Increased absorption and higher blood

DRUGS AFFECTED	DRUGS WHICH INTERACT	RESULT OF INTERACTION
		levels of levodopa. Metoclopramide can produce extra-pyramidal effects but does not seem to antagonize the effect of levodopa.
	Anticholinergic drugs, e.g. propantheline benzhexol benztropine	Reduced absorption and lower plasma concentration of levodopa. Clinical importance unknown.
	Pyridoxine (present in many proprietary multivitamin preparations.	Antagonism. Probably due to increased peripheral metabolism of levodopa. (Pyridoxine has no effect if a dopa decarboxylase inhibitor, e.g. carbidopa, is used.)
	Iron salts	Reduced absorption.
Bromocriptine Lysuride	Antipsychotic drugs	Antagonism.
Selegiline	Pethidine	Hyperpyrexia and CNS toxicity have been reported.

Anticholinesterases

| Neostigmine Pyridostigmine | Aminoglycosides Chloroquine Clindamycin Colistin Lincomycin | Antagonism. |

DRUGS AFFECTED	DRUGS WHICH INTERACT	RESULT OF INTERACTION
	Lithium Polymyxin Procainamide Propafenone Propranolol Quinidine	

DRUGS USED IN ANAESTHESIA

Anaesthetics

DRUGS AFFECTED	DRUGS WHICH INTERACT	RESULT OF INTERACTION
All	Antihypertensive drugs	Potentiation of hypotensive effect.
	Beta-adrenoceptor antagonists	Potentiation of hypotensive effect. Loss of compensatory reflex tachycardia.
	Chlorpromazine	Potentiation of hypotensive effect. Vasopressors ineffective because chlorpromazine blocks alpha-receptors.
Halothane Cyclopropane Trichlorethylene	Adrenaline Isoprenaline	These anaesthetics increase the sensitivity of the myocardium to sympathomimetie amines. Cardiac arrhythmias may occur.
	Levodopa	Increased risk of cardiac arrhythmias due to dopamine. Levodopa should be stopped 12 h before surgery.

DRUGS AFFECTED	DRUGS WHICH INTERACT	RESULT OF INTERACTION
Thiopentone	Sulphonamides	Thiopentone is displaced from protein binding. A smaller dose may be required.

Muscle relaxants

DRUGS AFFECTED	DRUGS WHICH INTERACT	RESULT OF INTERACTION
All	Colistin Polymyxin Procainamide Quinidine Lithium Propranolol (large doses)	Increased or prolonged paralysis. These drugs have neuromuscular blocking activity. Not reversed by neostigmine.

Competitive neuro-muscular blockers, e.g.
   tubocurarine
   gallamine
   pancuronium
	Aminoglycoside antibiotics
	Magnesium salts
	Clindamycin
	Lincomycin
	Nifedipine
	Verapamil
		Increased neuro-muscular block. Partially reversed by neostigmine and calcium.

	Diuretics Carbenoxolone	Potentiation by hypokalaemia is a probable but poorly documented risk.
Depolarizing neuromuscular blockers, e.g. suxamethonium	Neostigmine Pyridostigmine Ecothiopate eye-drops Cyclophosphamide Thiotepa	Potentiation and prolonged paralysis. These drugs have anticholinesterase activity.
	Digoxin	Increased risk of arrhythmias.

DRUGS AFFECTED	DRUGS WHICH INTERACT	RESULT OF INTERACTION

DRUGS USED IN INFECTIONS

DRUGS AFFECTED	DRUGS WHICH INTERACT	RESULT OF INTERACTION
Penicillins Cephalosporins	Probenecid	Delayed excretion and increased blood levels.
Phenoxymethyl-penicillin	Neomycin Guar gum	Reduced absorption.
Pivampicillin	Antacids	Reduced absorption.
Cephalothin and possibly other cephalosporins	Loop diuretics, e.g. frusemide Vancomycin Aminoglycosides	Increased risk of nephrotoxicity—especially if renal function is already impaired.
Tetracyclines (all)	Oral iron preparations Calcium, magnesium and aluminium salts Quinapril Zinc sulphate Sucralfate	Absorption reduced by chelation.
Cefamandole	Alcohol	'Antabuse-like' reaction.
Doxycycline	Barbiturates Phenytoin Carbamazepine	Reduced plasma concentration due to increased metabolism. Once-daily dosage is likely to be inadequate.
Aminoglycosides	Amphotericin Cephalothin Cyclosporin NSAIDs	Increased risk of nephrotoxicity.

DRUGS AFFECTED	DRUGS WHICH INTERACT	RESULT OF INTERACTION
	Loop diuretics	Increased risk of ototoxicity.
	Cisplatin Vancomycin	Increased risk of ototoxicity and nephrotoxicity.
Chloramphenicol	Phenobarbitone Rifampicin	Reduced plasma concentration.
Lincomycin	Kaolin mixtures	Reduced absorption.
Vancomycin	Cholestyramine	May inactivate vancomycin in bowel lumen.
Metronidazole	Alcohol	'Antabuse' reaction due to inhibition of aldehyde dehydrogenase.
	Cimetidine	Increased plasma concentration due to inhibition of metronidazole metabolism.
	Phenobarbitone	Increased metabolism and lower plasma concentration of metronidazole.
	Disulfiram	Acute psychotic reactions have been reported.
Quinolones, e.g. ciprofloxacin enoxacin	Antacids Sucralfate Iron salts Zinc salts	Reduced absorption.

DRUGS AFFECTED	DRUGS WHICH INTERACT	RESULT OF INTERACTION
Nalidixic acid Cinoxacin Nitrofurantoin	Probenecid	Delayed renal excretion and increased plasma concentration.
Isoniazid	Rifampicin	The risk of hepatotoxicity may be increased.
	Antacids	Reduced absorption of isoniazid.
Rifampicin	Antacids	Reduced absorption of rifampicin.
Griseofulvin	Phenobarbitone	Increased metabolism and lower plasma concentration of griseofulvin.
Miconazole	Amphotericin	Antagonism *in vitro*. Clinical importance unknown but they should not be used together.
Amphotericin	Aminoglycosides Cephalothin Cyclosporin	Increased risk of nephrotoxicity.
Ketoconazole Itraconazole	Antacids H_2-antagonists	Absorption depends on gastric acidity. May be reduced.
	Phenytoin Rifampicin	Increased metabolism and lower plasma concentration.
Fluconazole	Rifampicin	Reduced plasma concentration.

DRUGS AFFECTED	DRUGS WHICH INTERACT	RESULT OF INTERACTION
Acyclovir	Probenecid	Reduced renal excretion and increased plasma concentration.
Zidovudine	Probenecid	Increased plasma concentration and risk of toxicity.
Dapsone	Probenecid	Reduced renal excretion—increased risk of haemolytic anaemia.
Quinine	Cimetidine	Increased plasma concentration.
Chloroquine Hydroxychloroquine	Antacids	Reduced absorption.
	Cimetidine	Increased plasma concentration.
Mefloquine	Quinine Quinidine	Increased risk of side-effects.

DRUGS ACTING ON THE ENDOCRINE SYSTEM

Corticosteroids: dexamethasone hydrocortisone prednisone prednisolone	Diuretics: thiazides loop diuretics Carbenoxolone	Increased potassium loss and hypokalaemia.
	Carbamazepine Phenobarbitone Phenytoin Primidone Rifampicin	Increased metabolism and reduced therapeutic effect. Larger doses may be needed.

DRUGS AFFECTED	DRUGS WHICH INTERACT	RESULT OF INTERACTION
Dexamethasone	Aminoglutethimide	Increased metabolism and reduced effect.
Thyroxine	Cholestyramine	Reduced absorption.
	Carbamazepine Phenytoin Phenobarbitone Primidone Rifampicin	Increased thyroxine metabolism. May increase thyroxine requirements in patients with primary hypothyroidism.
Oral contraceptives	Barbiturates Carbamazepine Phenytoin Primidone Rifampicin Griseofulvin	Increased oestrogen and progestogen metabolism. Breakthrough bleeding and pregnancy may occur, especially with low-dose oestrogen preparations.
	Antibiotics, e.g. ampicillin tetracycline	Some oral antibiotics may increase oestrogen elimination by interfering with its enterohepatic circulation. Contraceptive failure has been reported but the risk is probably small.
	Ascorbic acid (vitamin C)	Inhibition of metabolism and increased plasma concentration of ethinyloestradiol.

DRUGS AFFECTED	DRUGS WHICH INTERACT	RESULT OF INTERACTION
	Anticonvulsants Methotrexate Trimethoprim Pyrimethamine Sulphasalazine	Possible risk of increased antifolate effect. Oral contraceptives can, rarely, cause folate deficiency.
Bromocriptine	Domperidone Metoclopramide	May antagonize hypoprolactinaemic effect.
	Erythromycin	Increased plasma concentration.
	Antipsychotic drugs	Antagonism of hypoprolactinaemic and antiparkinsonian effects.

DRUGS USED IN DIABETES

Insulin and oral antidiabetic drugs	Alcohol Monoamine oxidase inhibitors	Hypoglycaemia potentiated and prolonged.
	Beta-adrenoceptor antagonists	Hypoglycaemia may be potentiated and prolonged, and warning signs such as tremor masked.
	Corticosteroids, ACTH Diuretics: thiazides frusemide bumetanide Diazoxide Oral contraceptives	These drugs impair glucose tolerance and may produce hyperglycaemia. They antagonize antidiabetic drugs.

DRUGS AFFECTED	DRUGS WHICH INTERACT	RESULT OF INTERACTION
	Lithium	Lithium has complex effects on carbohydrate metabolism and may affect control of diabetes.
	Bezafibrate Clofibrate Gemfibrozil	May improve glucose tolerance and have an additive effect.
Sulphonylureas: chlorpropamide tolbutamide acetohexamide glibenclamide glymidine (not documented with others but caution advised)	Azapropazone Chloramphenicol Clofibrate Co-trimoxazole Fluconazole Miconazole Phenylbutazone Sulphaphenazole Sulphinpyrazone Trimethoprim	Potentiation of hypoglycaemia, mainly due to inhibition of sulphonylurea metabolism. Azapropazone, phenylbutazone and sulphaphenazole also displace tolbutamide from protein binding.
	Rifampicin	Increased metabolism of chlorpropamide, tolbutamide, glymidine and possibly others. A reduced effect should be anticipated.
	Nifedipine	May occasionally impair glucose tolerance and affect diabetic control.
Chlorpropamide	Thiazide + potassium-sparing diuretic	Increased risk of hyponatraemia.

DRUGS AFFECTED	DRUGS WHICH INTERACT	RESULT OF INTERACTION
	Alcohol	Flushing in some patients.
Metformin	Alcohol	Increased risk of lactic acidosis.
	Cimetidine	Increased plasma concentrations due to inhibition of renal excretion.

CYTOTOXIC AND IMMUNOSUPPRESSANT DRUGS

Mercaptopurine Azathioprine	Allopurinol	Potentiation and increased toxicity due to inhibition of metabolism by xanthine oxidase.
Methotrexate	Aspirin NSAIDs Probenecid	Decreased renal excretion may increase toxicity.
	Anticonvulsants Co-trimoxazole Trimethoprim Pyrimethamine Sulphasalazine	Possible risk of increased antifolate effect.
	Etretinate	Increased plasma concentration.
Cyclophosphamide	Chloramphenicol	Metabolism of cyclophosphamide to its active metabolites is inhibited. A reduced effect should be anticipated.

DRUGS AFFECTED	DRUGS WHICH INTERACT	RESULT OF INTERACTION
	Allopurinol	Increased blood levels of active metabolites and increased risk of bone marrow depression.
Fluorouracil	Cimetidine	Increased plasma concentration.
Cisplatin	Aminoglycosides	Increased risk of nephrotoxicity and ototoxicity.
Procarbazine	Alcohol	'Antabuse-like' reaction due to inhibition of aldehyde dehydrogenase.
Cyclosporin	Danazol Diltiazem Erythromycin Itraconazole Ketoconazole Nicardipine Progestogens Verapamil	Increased plasma concentration due to inhibition of cyclosporin metabolism.
	Phenytoin Phenobarbitone Rifampicin Carbamazepine	Increased metabolism and lower plasma concentration of cyclosporin.
	ACE inhibitors Potassium salts Potassium-sparing diuretics	The risk of hyperkalaemia may be increased.

DRUGS AFFECTED	DRUGS WHICH INTERACT	RESULT OF INTERACTION
	Aminoglycosides Co-trimoxazole Quinolones, e.g. ciprofloxacin NSAIDs	Risk of nephrotoxicity may be increased.

MISCELLANEOUS DRUGS

DRUGS AFFECTED	DRUGS WHICH INTERACT	RESULT OF INTERACTION
Oral iron preparations	Tetracyclines Magnesium trisilicate Zinc salts	Reduced absorption of iron.
Zinc salts	Oral iron	Reduced absorption of zinc.
Calcium salts	Thiazide diuretics	Increased risk of hypercalcaemia.
	Biphosphonates	Reduced absorption.
Biphosphonates	Antacids	Reduced absorption.
	Aminoglycosides	Risk of severe hypocalcaemia.
Ergotamine	Erythromycin	Ergotism has been reported.
Acetazolamide	Aspirin	Reduced excretion and risk of toxicity.
Terfenadine	Ketoconazole	Inhibition of metabolism and risk of cardiac toxicity.

Drug interactions with alcohol

DRUGS WHICH INTERACT	RESULT OF INTERACTION
Hypnotics and sedatives, antipsychotic drugs, antidepressants, opioid analgesics, antihistamines	The CNS depressant effect of alcohol is additive with that of all other sedatives. Alcohol increases the risk of death from overdose of CNS depressants.
Baclofen	Increased sedative effect.
Antipsychotic drugs	Exacerbation of extrapyramidal side-effects has been reported.
Antihypertensive drugs	Increased postural hypotension due to vasodilator effect of alcohol.
Peripheral vasodilators: isoxsuprine thymoxamine tolazoline	Postural hypotension.
Antianginal drugs: nitrates calcium-channel blockers	Postural hypotension.
Disulfiram Metronidazole Nimorazole Tinidazole Procarbazine	Increase blood levels of acetaldehyde by inhibiting aldehyde dehydrogenase. This can cause flushing, tachycardia, headache, dizziness, nausea and vomiting (the 'Antabuse' reaction).
Monosulfiram	Sufficient may be absorbed after topical administration to produce an 'Antabuse' reaction (see above).

DRUGS WHICH INTERACT	RESULT OF INTERACTION
Chlorpropamide	Flushing in some patients, probably due to inhibition of acetaldehyde metabolism.
Cefamandole	An 'Antabuse-like' reaction has been reported.
Metformin	Increased risk of lactic acidosis.
Aspirin	Increased risk of gastrointestinal bleeding.
Warfarin	Increased anticoagulant effect. Loss of anticoagulant control with intermittent drinking.
Paracetamol	The risk of hepatotoxicity following an overdose is increased in chronic alcoholics.
Monoamine oxidase inhibitors: phenelzine tranylcypromine	Some alcoholic and dealcoholized drinks contain tyramine. Risk of hypertensive crisis.
Cimetidine	Inhibits the metabolism of alcohol. Increased blood levels and increased subjective assessment of introxication have been reported.
Bromocriptine	Tolerance to bromocriptine may be reduced by alcohol.

Drugs and driving

When a drug listed in the following table is prescribed, patients should be advised:
1 Not to drive for the first few days after starting treatment or after a change in dose, until they are familiar with any unwanted effects of the drug.
2 Never to drive after drinking alcohol.
3 That it is illegal to drive or be in charge of a vehicle when the ability to drive is impaired by drugs.

It is the doctor's duty to inform their patient of any possible effects that a drug may have on driving.

DRUG	SIDE-EFFECTS WHICH MAY AFFECT DRIVING	ADDITIVE EFFECT WITH ALCOHOL
Hypnotics and sedatives		
Barbiturates Chloral hydrate Chlormethiazole Dichloralphenazone	Sedation. The effect of a nightly dose may persist for much of the following day.	+++
Benzodiazepines: used as hypnotics	Sedation. The effect of a nightly dose of flurazepam or nitrazepam may persist for much of the following day. Lormetazepam and temazepam have a shorter duration of effect but may also impair morning driving.	+++
used for anxiety	Sedation. Clobazam appears to have less effect on performance than others.	++

used for premedication, e.g.
    diazepam
    lorazepam
    midazolam
	Sedation. Patients should be advised not to drive for at least 12 h.	+++

DRUG	SIDE-EFFECTS WHICH MAY AFFECT DRIVING	ADDITIVE EFFECT WITH ALCOHOL
Chlormezanone Hydroxyzine Meprobamate, e.g. in Equagesic	Sedation—usually mild.	++

Antipsychotic drugs

Phenothiazines Haloperidol Pimozide Fluspirilene Zuclopenthixol Flupenthixol Sulpiride Oxypertine	Sedation—more with chlorpromazine and thioridazine than others. Tolerance occurs, and the risk is greatest during the first 7–14 days after treatment. Extrapyramidal effects may interfere with driving.	+
Lithium	May impair psychomotor performance.	?

Antidepressants

Amitriptyline Doxepin Mianserin Trazodone Trimipramine	Sedation. Tolerance occurs and the risk is greatest during the first few days of treatment.	++
Dothiepin Imipramine Maprotiline	Sedation—less than with amitriptyline, etc.	++
Butriptyline Clomipramine Desipramine Nortriptyline	Sedation—usually mild.	+

DRUG	SIDE-EFFECTS WHICH MAY AFFECT DRIVING	ADDITIVE EFFECT WITH ALCOHOL
Monoamine oxidase inhibitors (MAOIs)	May be sedative or stimulant.	++

Stimulants and appetite suppressants

Amphetamines Diethylpropion	Increased risk-taking behaviour.	+++
Fenfluramine	Sedation.	+

Opioid analgesics

Diamorphine Morphine Pentazocine Pethidine, etc.	Sedation.	+++
Codeine Dextropropo-xyphene Dihydrocodeine	Sedation—less than with diamorphine, etc.	++

Anti-inflammatory analgesics

Indomethacin Phenylbutazone	May possibly impair psychomotor performance.	?

Anticonvulsants

Carbamazepine Phenytoin Phenobarbitone Primidone	Sedation. Probably little effect in patients on long-term treatment. N.B. Driving must be stopped if treatment is changed.	++

DRUG	SIDE-EFFECTS WHICH MAY AFFECT DRIVING	ADDITIVE EFFECT WITH ALCOHOL
Antihistamines		
	Sedation. Non-sedative antihistamines, e.g. terfenadine, should be used for patients who have to drive.	
Muscle relaxants		
Baclofen Dantrolene	Sedation. Muscle weakness.	+
Anaesthetics		
Used for minor outpatient surgery	Patients should not drive for 24–48 h after anaesthetic, depending on the drug, duration of anaesthesia and the patient's response.	
Antihypertensive drugs		
All	Hypotension. Patients should be advised not to drive at the beginning of treatment or when dosage is being increased.	++
Beta-adrenoceptor blocking drugs: propranolol pindolol (possibly others)	Sedation and fatigue. Psychomotor performance may be impaired in the early stages of treatment.	+
Methyldopa Clonidine Indoramin	Sedation. Caution during first few days of treatment.	+

DRUG	SIDE-EFFECTS WHICH MAY AFFECT DRIVING	ADDITIVE EFFECT WITH ALCOHOL
Antidiabetic drugs		
Insulin Sulphonylureas, e.g. chlorpropamide tolbutamide	Hypoglycaemia.	++
Mydriatic eye-drops		
Atropine Cyclopentolate Homatropine	Paralysis of accommodation; blurring of near vision. Pupillary dilatation increases dazzle.	–
Miscellaneous		
Hyoscine Cyproheptadine Ketotifen Pizotifen Cyproterone Procarbazine Thiabendazole Ciprofloxacin Dantrolene	Sedation.	++

The effect of food on drug absorption

Food delays gastric emptying and reduces the rate of absorption of many drugs. The total amount of drug absorbed may or may not be reduced. Drugs whose total absorption may be reduced include:

Penicillins: phenoxymethylpenicillin, ampicillin, bacampicillin, cloxacillin, flucloxacillin, pivampicillin.

Tetracyclines: all except doxycycline and minocycline. (N.B. The absorption of all tetracyclines is reduced by dairy products.)

Erythromycin
Lincomycin
Rifampicin
Isoniazid
Captopril
Methotrexate (absorption reduced by milk products)
Penicillamine
Propantheline
Sotalol (absorption reduced by milk products)
Thyroxine

These drugs are best given at least 30 min before food.

Disodium etidronate—no food should be taken for 2 h before or after the drug.

Drugs whose absorption is delayed by food, with little effect on total absorption include:

Aspirin	Digoxin	Cephalexin
Paracetamol	Bumetanide	Cephradine
Barbiturates	Frusemide	(probably many others)

These drugs should be given on an empty stomach only if an immediate effect is required. Delayed absorption is not otherwise a disadvantage.

For a few drugs the absorption is increased by food. The importance of this is unknown. They include:

Griseofulvin (absorption increased by fatty foods)	Metoprolol
Nitrofurantoin	Propranolol
Spironolactone	Labetalol
Hydralazine	

These drugs should be taken in constant relation to food. Slow-release formulations are not affected.

Drug prescribing in renal failure

This section covers the following topics:
1 Drugs requiring dose reduction in renal failure.
2 Drugs to avoid altogether in renal failure.
3 Other drugs which may be harmful to patients with renal failure.
4 Drugs which are ineffective or less effective in renal failure.

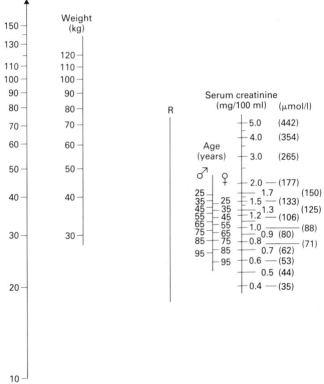

Nomogram for rapid evaluation of endogenous-creatinine clearance
With a ruler, join weight to age. Keep ruler at crossing-point of line marked R.
Then move the right-hand side of the ruler to the appropriate serum-creatinine
value and read the patient's clearance from the left side of the nomogram.

DRUGS REQUIRING DOSE REDUCTION IN RENAL FAILURE

Drugs eliminated entirely or partly by renal excretion accumulate in renal failure and smaller doses must be used. The extent of dose reduction depends on:

1 Whether the drug is eliminated entirely by excretion or is partly metabolized.

2 The toxicity of the drug, and whether this is related to the amount of drug present in the body. A smaller dose will result in toxic amounts in renal failure than in normal renal function.

3 The safety margin (therapeutic ratio) of the drug.

Increased sensitivity to some drugs occurs in renal failure for reasons other than impaired excretion and this may necessitate dose reduction.

In the following tables drugs are classified by body system. Renal impairment is divided into three categories of severity:

	Approximate GFR (ml/min)	Approximate serum creatinine (μmol/l)
1 Mild	20–50	150–300
2 Moderate	10–20	300–700
3 Severe	<10	<700

The serum creatinine concentration is only a rough guide to renal function because the value also depends on age, weight and sex. In particular it may be normal in elderly patients despite the fact that glomerular filtration rate falls with increasing age. The dose of drugs requiring dose reduction even in mild renal failure should be reduced in all patients aged over 60 years, whatever the value of the serum creatinine concentration.

Glomerular filtration rate can be estimated from serum creatinine, weight, age and sex, using a nomogram (see Figure, p. 50). More detailed information about dosage regimens can be found in the manufacturers' data-sheets.

DRUG	DEGREE OF RENAL IMPAIRMENT	COMMENTS
Gastrointestinal system		
Magnesium salts	2	Avoid. Risk of magnesium toxicity. Magnesium trisilicate also contains 6 mmol/10 ml sodium.
Aluminium-containing antacids Sucralfate	3	Aluminium may accumulate.
Gaviscon	3	Avoid. Contains 6 mmol/10 ml sodium.
Carbenoxolone	3	Avoid. Produces fluid retention.
Cimetidine	2 3	Reduce dose. Avoid. May produce confusional states.
Ranitidine	3	Reduce dose.
Famotidine	2	Reduce dose.
Metoclopramide	3	Avoid. Increased risk of extrapyramidal reactions.
Domperidone	3	Reduce dose.
Cisapride	3	Reduce dose.
Sulphasalazine	3	Risk of toxicity— rashes and blood dyscrasias.
Mesalazine	1	Avoid. Nephrotoxic.

DRUG	DEGREE OF RENAL IMPAIRMENT	COMMENTS
Fybogel	3	Avoid. High sodium content.

Cardiovascular system

DRUG	DEGREE OF RENAL IMPAIRMENT	COMMENTS
Digoxin	1	Reduce dose.
Diuretics:		
thiazides	2	Avoid. Ineffective.
bumetanide, frusemide	2	May need high doses.
ethacrynic acid	3	Avoid. Ototoxic.
potassium-sparing agents	1	Increased risk of hyperkalaemia.
	2	Avoid.
Antiarrhythmic drugs:		
disopyramide	1	Reduce dose.
flecainide	1	Reduce dose.
tocainide	1	Reduce dose.
procainamide	1	Avoid.
amiodarone	2	Iodine may accumulate. Increased risk of thyroid dysfunction.
Beta-blockers: acebutolol betaxolol metoprolol propranolol bisoprolol	3	Start with a small dose. Increased blood levels. May reduce renal blood flow.
atenolol nadolol pindolol sotalol	2	Reduce dose. Eliminated by renal excretion.
Xamoterol	2	Reduce dose. Eliminated by renal excretion.

DRUG	DEGREE OF RENAL IMPAIRMENT	COMMENTS
Antihypertensive drugs: bethanidine debrisoquine guanethidine	2	Avoid. Reduce renal blood flow and high risk of postural hypotension.
ACE inhibitors	1	Reduce dose. Increased toxicity and risk of hyperkalaemia.
hydralazine	3	Start with a small dose.
prazosin	3	Start with a small dose.
methyldopa	3	Start with a small dose.
diazoxide	3	Reduce dose.
Nifedipine Nicardipine	2	Start with a small dose.
Clofibrate	1–2	Reduce dose.
Bezafibrate	3	Avoid. Increased risk of myopathy and deterioration in renal function.
Gemfibrozil	3	Reduce dose.
Acipimox	1	Reduce dose.

Central nervous system

Hypnotics and sedatives	2	Start with a small dose. Increased sedation and CNS side-effects.

DRUG	DEGREE OF RENAL IMPAIRMENT	COMMENTS
Antipsychotic drugs	3	Start with a small dose. Increased risk of extrapyramidal effects.
Sulpiride	2	Avoid or reduce dose.
Lithium	1	Reduce dose. Avoid if possible.
	2	Avoid.
Antidepressants: fluoxetine	2	Reduce dose.
	3	Avoid.
fluvoxamine paroxetine	2	Reduce dose.
Analgesics: aspirin	3	Avoid. Increased risk of bleeding.
Solpadeine	3	Avoid. High sodium content.
NSAIDs	1	Avoid if possible. May cause fluid retention and deterioration in renal function.
azapropazone sulindac	2	Avoid. Excreted by the kidney.
diflunisal	3	Avoid. Excreted by the kidney.
codeine dihydrocodeine morphine	2	Avoid. Increased and prolonged effect.

DRUG	DEGREE OF RENAL IMPAIRMENT	COMMENTS
dextropropoxyphene (co-proxamol) pethidine	3	Avoid. CNS toxicity.
Ergotamine	2	Avoid. Risk of further deterioration in renal function.
Anticonvulsants: phenobarbitone primidone	3	Reduce dose. Increased sedation.
vigabatrin	1	Reduce dose.
Amantadine	1	Avoid. Excreted by the kidney.
Baclofen	1	Reduce dose. Excreted by the kidney.

Drugs used for infections

DRUG	DEGREE OF RENAL IMPAIRMENT	COMMENTS
Penicillins: benzylpenicillin	3	Reduce dose. Neurotoxic.
amoxycillin ampicillin	3	Reduce dose. Rashes more common.
bacampicillin pivampicillin talampicillin	3	Avoid.
co-amoxiclav Timentin	2	Reduce dose.
azlocillin carbenicillin piperacillin	2	Reduce dose.

DRUG	DEGREE OF RENAL IMPAIRMENT	COMMENTS
mezlocillin	3	Reduce dose.
Aztreonam	2	Reduce dose.
Cephalosporins: cefamandole cefoxitin ceftazidime ceftizoxime cefuroxime cephazolin cephradine	1	Reduce dose.
cefadroxil cefixime cefsulodin	2	Reduce dose.
cephalexin	3	Reduce dose.
cephalothin	1	Avoid. Nephrotoxic.
Aminoglycosides: all except neomycin	1	Reduce dose. Ototoxic and nephrotoxic.
neomycin	1	Avoid. Ototoxic and nephrotoxic.
Chloramphenicol	3	Avoid unless no alternative. Bone marrow depression.
Tetracyclines (except doxycycline and minocycline)	1	Avoid. Increase blood urea. Further deterioration in renal function.
Colistin	1	Reduce dose. Nephrotoxic and neurotoxic.

DRUG	DEGREE OF RENAL IMPAIRMENT	COMMENTS
Co-trimoxazole Trimethoprim	3	Reduce dose. Rashes and blood dyscrasias. Possible deterioration in renal function.
Vancomycin	1	Avoid if possible. Ototoxic and nephrotoxic.
Lincomycin	2	Use clindamycin instead.
Sulphonamides	2	Ensure high fluid intake. Rashes and blood dyscrasias.
Cinoxacin Nalidixic acid	2	Avoid. Nausea and rashes.
Nitrofurantoin	1	Avoid. Peripheral neuropathy. Pulmonary toxicity.
Ciprofloxacin Enoxacin Norfloxacin	2	Reduce dose.
Ofloxacin	1	Reduce dose.
Antituberculous drugs: capreomycin	1	Reduce dose. Ototoxic. Neurotoxic.
cycloserine	1	Avoid.
ethambutol	1	Reduce dose. Optic nerve damage.

DRUG	DEGREE OF RENAL IMPAIRMENT	COMMENTS
isoniazid	3	Reduce dose. Peripheral neuropathy.
Antifungal drugs: amphotericin	1	Use only if no alternative.
fluconazole	1	Reduce dose for multiple dose therapy.
flucytosine	1	Reduce dose.
terbinafine	1	Reduce dose.
acyclovir	1	Reduce dose.
Proguanil	3	Avoid. Haematological toxicity.
Piperazine	3	Reduce dose. Neurotoxic.
Zidovudine	1	Reduce dose. Increased risk of toxicity.
Endocrine system		
Insulin	3	May need dose reduction.
Acetohexamide Chlorpropamide	1	Avoid.
Other sulphonylureas	3	May need dose reduction. Increased risk of prolonged hypoglycaemia.

DRUG	DEGREE OF RENAL IMPAIRMENT	COMMENTS
Metformin	1	Avoid. Increased risk of lactic acidosis.
Propylthiouracil	1	Reduce dose.
Disodium etidronate	1 2	Reduce dose. Avoid. Excreted by kidney.
Clodronate	2	Avoid.

Cytotoxic and immunosuppressant drugs

Methotrexate	1 2	Reduce dose. Avoid. Nephrotoxic.
Cisplatin	1	Avoid if possible. Nephrotoxic.
Idarubicin	1	Reduce dose.
Bleomycin Cyclophosphamide Ifosfamide Melphalan Mercaptopurine Procarbazine Thioguanine	2	Reduce dose.
Azathioprine	3	Reduce dose.

Musculoskeletal and joint disease

Chloroquine	1	Reduce dose.
Hydroxychloroquine	3	Avoid prolonged use.
Gold salts	1	Avoid. Nephrotoxic.

DRUG	DEGREE OF RENAL IMPAIRMENT	COMMENTS
Penicillamine	1	Avoid or reduce dose. Nephrotoxic.
Allopurinol	2	Reduce dose. Increased toxicity.
Colchicine	3	Avoid or reduce dose. Increased toxicity.
Probenecid Sulphinpyrazone	2	Avoid. Ineffective.
Baclofen	1	Reduce dose. Excreted by kidney.

Drugs used in anaesthesia

Gallamine	2	Avoid. Prolonged paralysis.
Alcuronium Pancuronium Tubocurarine	2	Reduce dose. Prolonged paralysis.

Miscellaneous drugs

Potassium supplements Salt substitutes Potassium citrate	2	Avoid. Inability to excrete a potassium load. Risk of hyperkalaemia.
Sandocal	3	Avoid. High potassium content.
Acetazolamide	1	Avoid. Produces a metabolic acidosis.
Etretinate Isotretinoin	1	Avoid. Increased toxicity.

DRUG	DEGREE OF RENAL IMPAIRMENT	COMMENTS
Ephedrine Pseudoephedrine	3	Avoid. Increased CNS toxicity.
Vitamin A	3	Increases the already high vitamin A concentration in chronic renal failure. Hypervitaminosis A may contribute to hypercalcaemia.

Drug prescribing in liver disease

Liver disease takes many forms and it is unlikely that the effect on the response to drugs is the same in all.

In this section a brief discussion of the ways in which liver disease may alter the response to drugs is followed by a list of problems to anticipate when using particular drugs.

THE EFFECTS OF LIVER DISEASE ON RESPONSE TO DRUGS

Parenchymal liver disease

The liver is the main route of elimination for many drugs. Most are metabolized to inert substances which are then excreted in the bile or urine; a few (e.g. rifampicin) are excreted unchanged in the bile. In contrast to the creatinine clearance rate in renal disease, there is no simple test for hepatic function and routine liver function tests do not accurately reflect the capacity of the liver to metabolize drugs. Also the drug metabolizing reserve of the liver appears to be large for most drugs, and liver disease probably has to be severe before drug metabolism is impaired.

In patients with active liver disease or decompensated chronic liver disease (hypoalbuminaemia, raised bilirubin level, prolonged prothrombin time, encephalopathy) the metabolism of many drugs may be impaired. However, this is poorly correlated with severity of disease and in the individual patient the degree of impairment is unpredictable. Problems are most likely to occur with those drugs metabolized by the liver which have a low therapeutic ratio, e.g. phenytoin.

Portal–systemic shunting

After oral administration some drugs (e.g. propranolol, chlormethiazole) are extensively metabolized during their first passage through the liver such that less than 50% of an oral dose reaches the systemic circulation. Portacaval shunting can greatly increase the amount reaching the systemic circulation even if liver function is normal. The oral dose of these drugs should be reduced in patients with portacaval shunts and in patients with cirrhosis, in whom intrahepatic shunting is common.

Biliary obstruction

It is unlikely that biliary obstruction affects the elimination of drugs excreted into the bile because these are all water soluble and can be excreted in the urine instead.

Reduced protein binding of drugs

The hypoalbuminaemia of severe chronic liver disease is associated with reduced protein binding of several drugs. This may give rise to increased toxicity.

Cerebral sensitivity

In severe liver disease there is increased sensitivity to drugs acting on the central nervous system. This is independent of a reduced rate of metabolism of these drugs, but the precise mechanism is unknown. It can result in the precipitation of hepatic encephalopathy.

Impaired renal function

In severe liver disease the glomerular filtration rate falls and the elimination of drugs excreted by the kidney is reduced (see p. 51).

Fluid overload

Drugs that can produce fluid retention may exacerbate oedema and ascites in severe liver disease.

Other effects of liver disease on response to drugs are mentioned under the individual drugs.

THE USE OF HEPATOTOXIC DRUGS

Hepatotoxicity due to drugs can be predictable (dose related) or unpredictable (idiosyncratic).

There is no evidence that the risk of idiosyncratic hepatotoxicity is increased in patients with liver disease, but drugs producing dose-related hepatotoxicity should be avoided if possible as toxicity may occur at a lower dose than in patients with normal liver function.

An important reason for avoiding all hepatotoxic drugs is that, if they do produce jaundice in a patient with liver disease, it may be impossible to tell whether this is drug induced or due to deterioration of the original disease.

DRUG EFFECTS

In the following tables drugs are arranged by body system and pharmacological group.

DRUG	EFFECTS
Gastrointestinal system	
Antacids	Avoid those causing constipation, i.e. aluminium and calcium salts. Constipation increases the risk of encephalopathy in decompensated liver disease. In patients with fluid retention avoid those containing large amounts of sodium, e.g. magnesium trisilicate, Gaviscon.
Carbenoxolone	Produces fluid retention and hypokalaemia. Hypokalaemia may precipitate coma. Avoid in decompensated liver disease.
Cimetidine Ranitidine	Reduce dose. Occasional risk of confusional states.
Omeprazole	Reduce dose.
Metoclopramide	Reduce dose in severe liver disease.
Lomotil	Contains diphenoxylate (an opiate) and may precipitate coma in decompensated liver disease.
Chenodeoxycholic acid	Avoid in patients with chronic liver disease.

DRUG   EFFECTS

Cardiovascular system

Diuretics:
  thiazides
  loop diuretics
	Hypokalaemia may precipitate encephalopathy. Secondary hyperaldosteronism increases the risk of hypokalaemia; in severe liver disease spironolactone and amiloride are more effective than potassium supplements in preventing it. Increased risk of hypomagnesaemia in alcoholic cirrhosis.

Lignocaine Mexiletine Tocainide Flecainide	Metabolism impaired in decompensated liver disease. Reduce dose.
Procainamide	Avoid or reduce dose.
Propranolol	Metabolism impaired in decompensated liver disease and by portal systemic shunting. A reduction in oral dose may be required. Most other beta-blockers are not affected to the same extent but may need smaller doses.
Labetalol	Avoid. Hepatotoxic.
Methyldopa	Avoid. Hepatotoxic.
Verapamil	Elimination is impaired. Increased blood levels after oral and IV administration. Reduce dose.
Amlodipine Diltiazem Isradipine Nifedipine Nicardipine	Elimination is impaired. Dose reduction may be necessary.
Oral anticoagulants, e.g. warfarin	Increased sensitivity due to decreased synthesis of clotting

DRUG	EFFECTS
phenindione	factors. Avoid, especially if prothrombin time is already prolonged.
Cholestyramine	Interferes with the absorption of fat-soluble vitamins. Vitamin K deficiency could increase the hypoprothrombinaemia which occurs in decompensated liver disease.
Bezafibrate Clofibrate Gemfibrozil	Avoid in severe liver disease.
Simvastatin	Avoid. Hepatotoxic.

Respiratory system

Theophylline	Elimination is impaired in severe liver disease. Reduce dose.
Cough mixtures	Avoid those containing an opiate (codeine, pholcodine) in decompensated liver disease.
Antihistamines	Avoid sedative ones. May precipitate coma.

NERVOUS SYSTEM

Hypnotics and sedatives	None are safe. All can precipitate coma, due partly to increased cerebral sensitivity and partly to slower elimination. If a sedative is needed, a small dose of a benzodiazepine can be used. The metabolism of diazepam and chlordiazepoxide is impaired but temazepam and oxazepam are metabolized normally and are probably the drugs of choice.

DRUG	EFFECTS
Chlormethiazole	Blood levels after oral administration are higher in severe liver disease. Reduce oral dose.
Phenothiazines	Avoid. May precipitate coma. Hepatotoxicity, especially with chlorpromazine.
Antidepressants: monoamine oxidase inhibitors	Avoid. May precipitate coma. Hepatotoxic.
tricyclic antidepressants	Preferable to MAOIs but sedative effects may be increased. Iprindole is hepatotoxic.
fluoxetine fluvoxamine paroxetine sertraline	Reduce dose in severe liver disease.
Anticonvulsants: phenytoin	Metabolism may be impaired in severe liver disease. Reduce dose to avoid toxicity.
phenobarbitone primidone	Increased cerebral sensitivity and impaired metabolism in severe liver disease. May precipitate coma.
sodium valproate	Avoid if possible. Hepatotoxicity and liver failure can occur.
Dantrolene	Avoid in active or chronic liver disease. Hepatotoxic.

Analgesics and drugs used in arthritis

Aspirin	Increased risk of gastrointestinal bleeding. Avoid.
Anti-inflammatory analgesics, e.g.	Increased risk of gastrointestinal bleeding. Fluid retention and

DRUG	EFFECTS
indomethacin ibuprofen	increased risk of acute renal failure in severe liver disease.
Paracetamol	Elimination is impaired and blood levels are higher in decompensated liver disease. The dose required to produce hepatotoxicity may be smaller in patients with liver disease.
Gold salts	Avoid in severe liver disease. Hepatotoxic.
Opioid analgesics, e.g. morphine pethidine dextropropoxyphene (co-proxamol)	Avoid. May precipitate encephalopathy. Increased bioavailability and higher blood levels occur after oral administration.
Ergotamine	The risk of ergotism may be increased in severe liver disease or in patients with portal–systemic shunts.

Drugs used in infection

Tetracyclines	Increased risk of deterioration in renal function. Large intravenous doses (1–2 g daily) carry a definite risk of hepatotoxicity and should be avoided.
Erythromycin	Risk of ototoxicity with high doses. Erythromycin estolate can cause cholestatic jaundice and should be avoided.
Chloramphenicol	Elimination is impaired. Increased risk of bone marrow depression. Avoid.
Clindamycin	Reduce dose.

DRUG	EFFECTS
Fusidic acid	Biliary excretion is reduced. The risk of hepatotoxicity may be greater.
Metronidazole	Reduce dose in severe liver disease.
Isoniazid	Plasma half-life is prolonged in severe liver disease but this is likely to be important only in patients who are already slow acetylators of the drugs. Risk of hepatotoxicity may be increased in patients whose liver function is already impaired.
Rifampicin	Biliary excretion is impaired, blood levels are higher, and interference with bilirubin excretion is greater. The risk of hepatotoxicity is increased. Avoid or reduce dose in patients with severe liver disease.
Pyrazinamide	Avoid in severe liver disease. Hepatotoxic.
Niridazole	The incidence of CNS toxicity is increased in patients with cirrhosis or portal–systemic shunts.
Ketoconazole	Hepatotoxic. May accumulate in liver failure. Avoid if possible.

Drugs acting on the endocrine system

Corticosteroids	Side-effects are more common in chronic liver disease. Both impaired metabolism and reduced protein binding may contribute. Prednisone and cortisone are inactive until converted to prednisolone or hydrocortisone by the liver. Activation may be reduced in chronic liver disease and either prednisolone or hydrocortisone should be used.

DRUG	EFFECTS

Oral contraceptives
Oestrogens
Progestogens

They occasionally produce cholestatic jaundice and should not be given to patients with active liver disease or to women with a history of jaundice or itching in the last trimester of pregnancy.

Anabolic steroids, e.g.
  oxymetholone
  stanozolol

Produce dose-related cholestatic jaundice. Avoid.

Cyproterone acetate

Avoid. Dose-related hepatotoxicity.

Clomiphene

Avoid in severe liver disease.

Drugs used in diabetes

Sulphonylureas, e.g.
  chlorpropamide
  tolbutamide
  glibenclamide

Increased risk of hypoglycaemia. All can cause jaundice. Avoid.

Metformin

Risk of lactic acidosis is increased in liver disease. Avoid.

Drugs used in anaesthesia

Thiopentone

Reduced dose required for induction of anaesthesia—probably because protein binding is impaired.

Methohexitone

Avoid or reduce dose.

Suxamethonium

Prolonged apnoea may occur owing to reduced hepatic synthesis of pseudocholinesterase.

DRUG   EFFECTS

Malignant disease and immunosuppressants

Azathioprine   Immunosuppressive activity may be
                              reduced owing to impaired
                              conversion to active metabolite.
                              Bone marrow and liver toxicity are
                              probably caused by the unchanged
                              drug and the risk may be increased.

Methotrexate   Dose-related hepatotoxicity. Should
                              not be used for the treatment of
                              benign conditions (e.g. psoriasis) in
                              the presence of liver disease.

Doxorubicin   Reduce dose.
Epirubicin
Idarubicin

Miscellaneous

Etretinate   Avoid. May produce further
Isotretinoin   deterioration in liver function.

Drug prescribing for the elderly

The incidence of adverse drug reactions is increased in elderly patients, and this is at least partly due to age-related changes which affect the response to certain drugs:

1 Renal function declines with age, especially in sick elderly patients, and the clearance of drugs eliminated largely by the kidney is reduced. The serum creatinine level is not a good guide to renal function in the elderly because creatinine production also falls with age; but creatinine clearance can be estimated from the serum creatinine level by using the nomogram on p. 50. It is probably wise to assume that most sick elderly patients will have a GFR of 50 ml/min or less, and to reduce the dose of all drugs listed in Group 1 on pp. 51–62.

2 Drug metabolism is less predictably affected by age. It is reduced for some drugs but appears to be unchanged for others. The first-pass metabolism of some drugs is reduced and this may result in high peak blood levels after oral administration.

3 Lean body mass is reduced in some elderly patients and smaller doses will be needed to achieve the same dose per unit body-weight.

4 A fall in serum albumin concentration in some elderly patients reduces the protein binding of some drugs but the clinical importance of this is uncertain.

5 Other changes occurring with age may affect the sensitivity to a drug independently of changes in its pharmacokinetics. For example, the elderly are more sensitive to drugs acting on the central nervous system, and impaired cardiovascular homoeostasis is thought to account for their increased susceptibility to drugs, causing postural hypotension. They are also more likely to develop side-effects such as urine retention, constipation and hypothermia.

6 Drug interactions are more likely to occur in the elderly, partly because of the changes in drug elimination, protein binding and sensitivity listed above and partly because the elderly receive more drugs than the young.

Drugs which most commonly produce problems are listed in the following table.

DRUGS THAT MAY CAUSE PROBLEMS IN ELDERLY PATIENTS

See also Drugs in renal failure—Group 1, pp. 51–62.

DRUG   PROBLEMS AND COMMENTS

Alimentary system

Carbenoxolone	Increased risk of hypertension, oedema, heart failure and hypokalaemia. Avoid prolonged use of high dose.
Cimetidine Ranitidine	Renal excretion is reduced and blood levels are higher. Confusional states are more common. Reduce dose.
Metoclopramide	Increased risk of parkinsonism and of tardive dyskinesia. Avoid prolonged use.

Cardiovascular system

Digoxin	Renal excretion is reduced. Increased risk of toxicity. Reduce dose. Many patients in sinus rhythm or with slow atrial fibrillation do not need it. CNS toxicity is more common.
Diuretics: thiazides bumetanide frusemide piretanide	Dehydration, hyponatraemia, postural hypotension, incontinence and urine retention are more common. Avoid excessive diuresis. Poor diet may predispose to hypokalaemia. The effect of loop diuretics (frusemide, bumetanide) is reduced and larger doses may be needed.
amiloride spironolactone triamterene	Increased risk of hyperkalaemia.
thiazide/potassium-sparing combinations (Moduretic, Dyazide)	Risk of hyponatraemia. Avoid or use smallest dose.

DRUG	PROBLEMS AND COMENTS
acetazolamide	Renal excretion may be reduced. Reduce dose, especially if side-effects occur.
Beta-adrenoceptor antagonists	Bradycardia and precipitation of heart failure are more likely to occur—due mainly to underlying ischaemic heart disease. First-pass elimination of propranolol may be reduced and peak blood levels after oral administration increased. Atenolol, nadolol, pindolol and sotalol are excreted by the kidney and blood levels may be higher. Use small doses initially.
Antihypertensive drugs:	Postural hypotension is more common and may result in falls or stroke. Start with small doses and avoid rapid or excessive reduction in blood pressure.
bethanidine debrisoquine guanethidine	Avoid—severe postural hypotension common.
clonidine	Avoid—increased risk of inadvertent sudden withdrawal causing rebound hypertension.
ACE inhibitors, e.g. captopril enalapril	Increased risk of hypotension and renal impairment. Initial dose should be small.
Anticoagulants: heparin	Increased risk of bleeding. Avoid prolonged use of full anticoagulant doses.
warfarin	Increased anticoagulant effect. Start with smaller doses.

DRUG	EFFECTS

Respiratory system

Sympathomimetic bronchodilators	May be less effective due to reduced beta-receptor responsiveness. Clinical importance unknown.
Ephedrine (present in compound asthma preparations)	Urine retention.
Theophylline and derivatives, e.g. aminophylline	Blood levels may be higher and side-effects—anorexia, nausea, confusion—more common. Use small doses initially and increase gradually.

Nervous system

Hypnotics and sedatives:	Increased and prolonged effects. Daytime drowsiness, ataxia, falls, restlessness and confusion more common.
barbiturates	Avoid.
benzodiazepines	Use small doses, preferably of those with a short half-life, e.g. temazepam, lormetazapem.
chlormethiazole	Elimination is impaired and blood levels are higher. Use small doses.
Antipsychotic drugs, e.g. phenothiazines haloperidol	Extrapyramidal effects are more common and the risk of tardive dyskinesia is increased. Anticholinergic effects of phenothiazines—urine retention, constipation, dry mouth—are poorly tolerated. Postural hypotension may occur. Increased risk of hypothermia in winter. Use small doses.

DRUG	PROBLEMS AND COMMENTS
Tricyclic antidepressants	Elimination is impaired and blood levels are higher. Anticholinergic effects—urine retention, constipation, dry mouth—are poorly tolerated. Postural hypotension and confusional states are more common. Use small doses initially.
Mianserin	Elimination is impaired. The risk of neutropenia may be increased. Reduce dose.
Trazodone	Elimination is impaired. Increased sedation. Reduce dose.
Lithium	Reduced renal excretion. Usually need smaller doses. Polyuria can lead to dehydration and incontinence.
Phenytoin	Protein binding is reduced. The clinical importance of this is unknown but total blood levels used for monitoring therapy will be low in relation to the free concentration.
Drugs used for parkinsonism: levodopa bromocriptine	Side-effects, e.g. confusional states, psychotic and behavioural reactions, postural hypotension, are more common.
amantadine	Increased risk of confusion and hallucinations.
anticholinergic drugs, e.g. benzhexol benztropine	Anticholinergic effects—urine retention, constipation, dry mouth—are poorly tolerated. Confusional states may occur.
selegiline	Increased risk of amphetamine-like side-effects—agitation, confusion, etc.

DRUG   PROBLEMS AND COMMENTS

Analgesics

Opioid analgesics   Blood levels of pethidine,
                                 pentazocine, methadone and
                                 dextropropoxyphene (co-proxamol)
                                 are higher and side-effects—nausea,
                                 hypotension, CNS effects—are more
                                 common.

Benorylate   Reduce dose to avoid salicylate
                                 toxicity (tinnitus, etc.).

Anti-inflammatory   Fluid retention can interfere with
analgesics: treatment of heart failure and
  all   hypertension. Increased risk of renal
                                 impairment. The risk of
                                 gastrointestinal toxicity may be
                                 increased Avoid those with a long
                                 half-life, e.g. piroxicam.

  azapropazone   Blood levels are higher. Reduce dose.

  phenylbutazone   Blood levels are higher and side-
                                 effects more common. The risk of
                                 aplastic anaemia is probably
                                 increased. Avoid.

  indomethacin   Blood levels are higher and CNS
                                 side-effects—headache, lethargy,
                                 etc.—may be more common.

  mefenamic acid   Increased risk of renal failure,
                                 especially in patients also taking
                                 diuretics.

Antibacterial drugs

Tetracyclines   Reduced renal excretion. Side-
                                 effects—nausea and a rise in blood
                                 urea—are more common.

DRUG	PROBLEMS AND COMMENTS
Aminoglycosides, e.g. gentamicin tobramycin	Reduced renal excretion. Increased sensitivity to ototoxic effects. Use smaller doses and monitor blood levels.
Co-trimoxazole	Increased risk of blood dyscrasias.
Nitrofurantoin	Reduced renal excretion. Increased nausea and risk of peripheral neuropathy. Avoid if possible.

Endocrine system

Thyroxine	Elderly patients usually need smaller doses. In patients with ischaemic heart disease the initial replacement dose should not exceed 50 µg daily to avoid precipitating angina.
Oral hypoglycaemic agents	Increased risk of prolonged hypoglycaemia with sulphonylureas. A short-acting drug, e.g. tolbutamide, should be used. Avoid chlorpropamide.
Corticosteroids	Increased risk of osteoporosis and fractures, especially in postmenopausal women.

Drugs in pregnancy

Drugs given to a pregnant woman can harm the fetus at any time from the third week to the end of pregnancy. In the first week after conception, before implantation has occurred, it is probable that potentially harmful drugs have an all-or-none effect; either the embryo dies or the damaged cells are replaced by undifferentiated cells which develop normally. After implantation, differentiation of the embryo begins and continues for the next 8 weeks. Damage during this period of organogenesis (3rd–11th weeks of pregnancy) can produce congenital malformations. Later in pregnancy major malformations cannot be produced but drugs can still affect the growth and functional development of fetal tissues and organs.

The following tables do not include drugs that have been shown to harm the fetus in animals. The relevance of these observations to humans is unknown. They are listed in Appendix 4 of the *British National Formulary*.

DRUGS THAT CAN HARM THE FETUS IN THE FIRST TRIMESTER

DRUG	COMMENTS

Proven teratogens—high risk

DRUG	COMMENTS
Thalidomide	
Cytotoxic drugs	Alkylating agents, e.g. cyclophosphamide. Folate antagonists, e.g. methotrexate.
Etretinate	Pregnancy should be avoided for
Isotretinoin	1 year after stopping etretinate and 4 weeks after stopping isotretinoin.

Proven teratogens—low risk

Other cytotoxic drugs
Anticonvulsants
Warfarin
Lithium
Quinine (high doses)
Alcohol
Vitamin A (high doses)

DRUG	COMMENTS

Possible teratogens

Azathioprine

| Trimethoprim (co-trimoxazole) Pyrimethamine (Daraprim, Fansidar, Maloprim) Griseofulvin Flucytosine Penicillamine Podophyllum Diethylpropion | These drugs are folate antagonists. Folate supplements should be given. |

Oestrogens
Progestogens

| Live vaccines, e.g. rubella | Vaccination produces a viraemia and virus can be recovered from the fetus. However, the risk of malformation does not appear to be increased. |

Other effects

| Androgens Oestrogens Progestogens Danazol | Virilization of female fetus. The small doses in oral contraceptives are unlikely to have this effect. |

| Cyproterone acetate (Dianette) | Feminization of male fetus is a possibility. |

| Stilboestrol | High doses associated with development of carcinoma of vagina in female offspring 15–20 years later. |

| Diagnostic radiology | Increased risk of childhood leukaemia and (?) other neoplasms. |

| Streptokinase Urokinase | May cause premature separation of the placenta. |

ADVERSE EFFECTS ON THE FETUS AND NEONATE OF DRUGS GIVEN DURING THE SECOND AND THIRD TRIMESTERS

DRUG	ADVERSE EFFECTS

Gastrointestinal system

Sulphasalazine	Could produce neonatal haemolysis or methaemoglobinaemia, but these have not been reported. Folate supplements should be given to the mother.
Misoprostol	Increases uterine tone.

Cardiovascular system

Thiazide diuretics	Should not be used during the third trimester. They reduce plasma volume and placental perfusion and may cause neonatal thrombocytopenia.
Beta-adrenoceptor antagonists, e.g. propranolol oxprenolol atenolol sotalol	May aggravate or produce neonatal hypoglycaemia. Fetal and neonatal bradycardia may occur, especially in pregnancies already complicated by placental insufficiency (e.g. severe maternal hypertension).
Bethanidine Debrisoqine Guanethidine	Postural hypotension and reduced uteroplacental perfusion. Should not be used to treat hypertension in pregnancy.
ACE inhibitors	May adversely affect fetal and neonatal blood pressure control and renal function.

DRUG	ADVERSE EFFECTS
Diazoxide	Prolonged use can cause alopecia and impaired glucose tolerance in the neonate.
Minoxidil	Neonatal hirsutism has been reported.
Reserpine	Neonatal bradycardia, nasal stuffiness and drowsiness have been reported.
Amiodarone	Releases iodine and could possibly cause neonatal hypothyroidism.
Oral anticoagulants	Fetal or neonatal haemorrhage can occur. Subcutaneous heparin should be substituted in the last 3 weeks of pregnancy in patients with heart valve prostheses and can be substituted throughout for venous thromboembolism. (See also 'First trimester'.)
Streptokinase Urokinase	Risk of fetal haemorrhage.
Clofibrate and related drugs Simvastatin and related drugs	Theoretical risk of interference with fetal growth and development.

Respiratory system

Theophylline	Neonatal irritability, tachycardia and apnoea have been reported.
Iodides (present in some proprietary cough medicines)	Neonatal goitre and hypothyroidism have been reported.

DRUG   ADVERSE EFFECTS

Nervous system

Alcohol   Growth retardation and neonatal
                            withdrawal syndrome in babies of
                            alcoholic mothers. (See also 'First
                            trimester'.)

Hypnotics and sedatives   All can depress neonatal respiration.

Benzodiazepines   Neonatal hypotonia and
                            hypothermia have occurred after
                            large amounts of diazepam ($>30\,$mg)
                            given during labour. Regular use of
                            benzodiazepines during the last
                            weeks of pregnancy can produce
                            neonatal drowsiness and hypotonia
                            which may last for several days.
                            Neonatal withdrawal effects have
                            been reported occasionally.

Barbiturates   Neonatal withdrawal effects can
                            occur in babies born to mothers
                            taking regular barbiturates during
                            the last trimester.

Tricyclic antidepressants   Neonatal tachycardia, irritability,
                            tremor, muscle spasms and
                            convulsions have been reported.

Phenothiazines   Extrapyramidal effects in the
                            neonate have been reported.

Lithium   Fetal thyroid suppression may
                            produce neonatal goitre. Neonatal
                            lithium toxicity produces hypotonia
                            and cyanosis, and is usually
                            associated with poor control of
                            maternal lithium therapy. (See also
                            'First trimester'.)

Phenytoin   Inhibit the synthesis of vitamin K-
Phenobarbitone   dependent clotting factors. Neonatal
                            haemorrhage may occur.

DRUG	ADVERSE EFFECTS
	Prophylactic vitamin K$_1$ should be given to the mother before delivery and to the baby at birth. Neonatal withdrawal effects have been reported with phenobarbitone. (See also 'First trimester'.)
Anaesthetics	Depress neonatal respiration.
Local anaesthetics	Neonatal depression, hypotonia and bradycardia can follow the use of large doses for paracervical or epidural block. Prilocaine and procaine can produce methaemoglobinaemia.
Pyridostigmine Neostigmine	Large doses can produce neonatal myasthenia.

Analgesics and joint disease

Opioid analgesics	Depress neonatal respiration. Withdrawal effects occur in babies born to mothers dependent on narcotics. They have also been reported following prolonged therapeutic use of pentazocine, dextropropoxyphene and codeine.
Aspirin	Small doses interfere with platelet function and larger doses can also produce hypoprothrombinaemia. Neonatal haemorrhage can occur. Inhibition of fetal prostaglandin synthesis may cause closure of the ductus arteriosus *in utero*, with pulmonary hypertension and respiratory problems at birth. Displaces unconjugated bilirubin from protein binding and increases the risk of kernicterus in jaundiced infants, especially if premature. Avoid in the third trimester.

DRUG	ADVERSE EFFECTS

NSAIDs, e.g.
    indomethacin
    naproxen
	Inhibition of fetal prostaglandin synthesis as for aspirin (see above). Avoid if possible in the third trimester.

Penicillamine	Fetal abnormalities have been reported following use after the first trimester. Avoid if possible. (See also 'First trimester'.)
Ergotamine	Oxytocic effects on uterus.

Drugs used in infections

Tetracyclines	Deposited in developing bones and teeth. Discoloration of the deciduous teeth occurs from the 14th week, and the permanent teeth are affected during the last 3 months.

Aminoglycosides:
    streptomycin
    gentamicin
    tobramycin
    kanamycin
	May cause auditory or vestibular nerve damage. Deafness has been reported with streptomycin. Risk with gentamicin and tobramycin is probably small.

Chloramphenicol	The neonatal 'Grey syndrome' can occur in babies born to mothers given chloramphenicol at the end of pregnancy.

Sulphonamides, e.g.
    co-trimoxazole
    Fansidar
	May produce neonatal haemolysis and methaemoglobinaemia. Displace unconjugated bilirubin from protein binding and increase the risk of kernicterus in jaundiced infants, especially if premature.

Nitrofurantoin	May produce neonatal haemolysis.
Rifampicin	Risk of hypoprothrombinaemia and bleeding in the perinatal period may be increased.

DRUG	ADVERSE EFFECTS
Chloroquine	Neonatal chorioretinitis has been reported but the risk is probably small. (Chloroquine remains a drug of choice for the treatment of malaria in pregnancy.)
Primaquine	May produce neonatal haemolysis and methaemoglobinaemia.
Dapsone (Maloprim)	May produce neonatal haemolysis and methaemoglobinaemia. Folate supplements should be given to the mother because of low-grade haemolysis.

Endocrine system

Antithyroid drugs	Suppression of fetal thyroid function can produce neonatal goitre and hypothyroidism. Usually mild and transient. Dosage can usually be reduced towards the end of pregnancy.
Radioactive iodine	Damage to fetal thyroid, with permanent hypothyroidism.
Iodides	Neonatal goitre and hypothyroidism have been reported.
Corticosteroids	Doses not exceeding 10 mg prednisolone daily appear to be harmless. It is possible that higher doses could produce fetal and neonatal adrenal suppression.
Sulphonylureas, e.g. chlorpropamide tolbutamide	Neonatal hypoglycaemia may occur. If oral antidiabetic therapy is used, it should be stopped at least 3 days before delivery.
Androgens Oestrogens Progestogens Danazol	Virilization of female fetus. (See also 'First trimester'.)

DRUG	ADVERSE EFFECTS

Vitamins

Vitamin A	Excessive doses may be teratogenic.
Vitamin K analogues: menadiol sodium diphosphate (not vitamin K₁)	May produce neonatal haemolysis. Displaces unconjugated bilirubin from protein binding and increases the risk of kernicterus in jaundiced infants, especially if premature.

Skin

Podophyllum	Fetal death has been reported. Avoid application to large areas and anogenital warts. (See also 'First trimester'.)
Povidone-iodine	Sufficient iodine may be absorbed to affect the fetal thyroid gland.

DRUGS WITH UNWANTED EFFECTS ON THE MOTHER

Calcium antagonists: diltiazem nifedipine nicardipine verapamil	Relax uterine smooth muscle and may inhibit labour.
Disopyramide	May induce labour.
Diazoxide	Inhibition of uterine activity may produce temporary cessation of labour.
Heparin	Osteoporosis has been reported after prolonged use.

DRUG	ADVERSE EFFECTS
Beta-sympathomimetic drugs, e.g. salbutamol terbutaline	Parenteral use in the management of premature labour produces: **1** A tachycardia which can precipitate heart failure in women with pre-existing cardiovascular disease. The risk is increased by corticosteroids, e.g. dexamethasone, which produce fluid retention. **2** An increase in blood sugar which can result in severe hyperglycaemia and ketosis in diabetic women. Parenteral use in the treatment of asthma could delay the onset of labour.
NSAIDs, e.g. aspirin indomethacin naproxen	Can delay the onset and increase the duration of labour by inhibiting prostaglandin synthesis.
Opioid analgesics	Produce gastric stasis and increase the risk of inhalation pneumonia occurring during labour.
Lithium	Renal clearance is increased during pregnancy and larger doses may be required. Toxicity may occur if the dose is not reduced after delivery.
Phenytoin	Maternal plasma total phenytoin concentrations may fall without a fall in free phenytoin concentration. This affects the interpretation of concentrations used for monitoring therapy.
Tetracyclines	Large doses (> 1 g daily) given intravenously can produce severe liver damage.
Erythromycin estolate	The risk of hepatotoxicity may be increased.

DRUG	ADVERSE EFFECTS
Corticosteroids	Steroid cover will be required during labour by women on regular corticosteroid therapy, or whose treatment has been withdrawn during the previous 2 months.

Smoking and pregnancy

Smoking during pregnancy is associated with a reduction in birth-weight and an increase in perinatal mortality rate. There is also some evidence that the risk of spontaneous abortion is increased in women who smoke.

Drugs and lactation

Most drugs taken by a lactating mother are excreted in her milk, but usually the amount will be too small to affect the baby. However, the elimination of many drugs is impaired in the neonatal period, and drugs taken regularly may accumulate and reach levels sufficient to produce an effect. The risk is increased by prematurity.

The drugs listed in the first table are excreted in breast milk in amounts that could produce unwanted effects in the baby, and in some cases have been shown to do so. Two further tables list drugs that are probably safe. There is insufficient information available to produce a comprehensive list, and absence of a drug from the first table does not mean that it is safe.

DRUGS THAT MAY BE HARMFUL

DRUG	ADVERSE EFFECTS ON CHILD
Gastrointestinal system	
Atropine	Evidence that atropine is present in breast milk is conflicting, but it could produce anticholinergic effects in the baby and is best avoided.

Anthraquinone laxatives:
  cascara
  danthron
	Evidence is conflicting but increased bowel activity in the baby has been reported. Senna is probably safe, but avoid large doses.

Sulphasalazine	Possible risk of haemolytic anaemia in G6PD-deficient babies.
Cardiovascular system	
Amiodarone	Present in milk in significant amounts. Theoretical risk of iodine-induced neonatal hypothyroidism.

DRUG	ADVERSE EFFECTS ON CHILD
Beta-adrenoceptor antagonists	Amounts in milk are probably too small to affect the baby, but could produce signs of beta-blockade: bradycardia, hypoglycaemia.
metoprolol oxprenolol propranolol	Very small amounts in milk— unlikely to affect baby at usual dose.
acebutolol atenolol nadolol sotalol	High concentrations have been found in milk. Bradycardia and hypoglycaemia could occur with therapeutic doses.
Labetalol	Amounts in milk are probably too small to affect the baby but could produce signs of beta-blockade: bradycardia, hypoglycaemia.
Anticoagulants	Risk of haemorrhage with phenindione. Warfarin and nicoumalone appear to be safe but it may be advisable to give the baby vitamin K_1. Heparin is not excreted in breast milk.

Respiratory system

Theophylline	Irritability has been reported in a breast-fed baby whose mother took 200 mg aminophylline every 6 h. Slow-release preparations are probably safe.
Ephedrine Pseudoephedrine	Irritability and disturbed sleep have been reported with ephedrine + brompheniramine. Significant amounts of pseudoephedrine in milk.
Antihistamines	Present in milk. Drowsiness and irritability have been reported with clemastine. (See also 'Ephedrine'.)

DRUG	ADVERSE EFFECTS ON CHILD

Nervous system

Alcohol	Large amounts can affect the baby.
Barbiturates	High doses can produce drowsiness.
Benzodiazepines	Drowsiness, lethargy and failure to thrive have been reported. Regular use of high doses should be avoided, but single doses are probably harmless. Those with a short half-life may be preferable to longer-acting drugs.
Chloral hydrate	Drowsiness.
Meprobamate (e.g. in Equagesic)	High concentrations in milk. Drowsiness.
Phenothiazines	Drowsiness has been reported with chlorpromazine, but amounts in milk of most phenothiazines are probably too small to be harmful.
Sulpiride	Significant amounts in milk. Avoid.
Lithium	Present in milk in amounts that can affect the baby, but the risk of toxicity—hypotonia, lethargy—is probably small if maternal blood levels are well controlled. It will be increased by dehydration, e.g. if the baby is ill or has diarrhoea. Many women on lithium have breast-fed their babies without complications but bottle-feeding is preferable.
Fluoxetine	Only small amounts in milk but could accumulate in the infant.
Phenobarbitone Primidone	Drowsiness could occur. Phenobarbitone in combination with phenytoin has been associated with a case of methaemoglobinaemia in one baby.

DRUG   ADVERSE EFFECTS ON CHILD

Analgesics and joint disease

Opioid analgesics, e.g.
   diamorphine
   morphine
   methadone
   pethidine
	Therapeutic doses are unlikely to affect the baby. Regular use of high doses can produce dependence and withdrawal effects. It appears to be safe for mothers on methadone maintenance to breast-feed their babies.

Aspirin	Regular use of large doses could impair platelet function and produce hypoprothrombinaemia if neonatal vitamin K stores are low. Metabolic acidosis has been reported.
Indomethacin	Significant amounts are present in milk. Convulsions have been reported in one breast-fed neonate.
Gold salts	Present in milk. Theoretical risk of toxicity.

Drugs used in infections

Aminoglycosides:
   gentamicin
   kanamycin
   streptomycin
   tobramycin
	Probably not absorbed by the baby. Alteration of bowel flora and diarrhoea are possible risks.

Chloramphenicol	Possibility of bone marrow depression. Amounts in milk probably too small to cause 'Grey syndrome'.
Tetracyclines	Absorption by the baby is probably prevented by chelation with milk calcium, and tooth discoloration is therefore unlikely.

DRUG	ADVERSE EFFECTS ON CHILD
Sulphonamides Co-trimoxazole	Risk of haemolytic anaemia in G6PD-deficient babies. Possible risk of kernicterus in jaundiced babies.
Metronidazole	Present in milk in significant amounts. Not known to be harmful but avoid for 24 h after large single dose.
Nalidixic acid	Amounts in milk appear to be too small to be harmful in normal babies but one case of haemolytic anaemia has been reported in a neonate whose mother was given nalidixic acid while breast-feeding.
Ciprofloxacin	High concentrations in breast milk.
Nitrofurantoin	Only small amounts in milk but could be enough to produce haemolysis in G6PD-deficient babies.
Isoniazid	Theoretical risk of convulsions and neuropathy. Prophylactic pyridoxine should be given to mother and baby.
Dapsone	Haemolytic anaemia can occur, especially in G6PD-deficient babies.
Antimalarials: Fansidar Maloprim	*See* sulphonamides, above. *See* dapsone, above.
Idoxuridine	May make milk taste unpleasant.

Endocrine system

Sulphonylureas	Little available information but theoretical risk of hypoglycaemia in the neonate.

DRUG	ADVERSE EFFECTS ON CHILD
Thyroxine	Amounts in milk too small to mask neonatal hypothyroidism but could possibly interfere with screening tests for hypothyroidism.
Antithyroid drugs: carbimazole propylthiouracil	Propylthiouracil is present in amounts which are probably too small to affect the baby. Amounts of carbimazole are also small but high doses could affect neonatal thyroid function.
Radioactive iodine	Hypothyroidism, which may be permanent. Breast-feeding is contraindicated.
Corticosteroids	Prolonged treatment with high doses (>10 mg prednisolone daily) could produce adrenal suppression but this has not been reported.
Oral contraceptives	Amounts of oestrogen and progestogen in milk are too small to affect the baby. Suppression of lactation is unlikely if the dose of oestrogen does not exceed 50 µg but some people prefer not to use combined oral contraceptives until lactation is well established (4–6 weeks postpartum). Progestogen-only contraceptives have no effect on lactation and may be preferred in the postpartum period.
Cyproterone acetate	Significant amounts in milk. Possible risk of antiandrogen effects on the baby.

DRUG	ADVERSE EFFECTS ON CHILD

Cytotoxics and immunosuppressants

All cytotoxics	Probably some risk of toxicity with most. Cyclophosphamide has caused neutropenia in a breast-fed baby. Breast-feeding is contraindicated.
Cyclosporin	Present in milk and potentially harmful. Breast-feeding best avoided.

Miscellaneous

Ergotamine	Ergotism—vomiting, diarrhoea, convulsions, circulatory disturbances.
Vitamin A	Prolonged use of large doses (> 4000 units daily) could possibly produce hypervitaminosis A in the baby.
Vitamin D	Prolonged use of large doses (> 500 units daily) could possibly produce neonatal hypercalcaemia.
Iodine (e.g. in cough mixtures containing iodides)	Concentrated in milk. Risk of neonatal hypothyroidism and goitre.
Povidone-iodine	Sufficient iodine can be absorbed from vaginal preparations to affect the baby's thyroid.
Etretinate Isotretinoin	Avoid.
Caffeine	Regular intake of large amounts could affect the baby.
Nicotine	Smoking more than 20 cigarettes a day may decrease lactation and cause jitteriness in the baby.

DRUGS PRESENT IN MILK IN SIGNIFICANT AMOUNTS, BUT NOT KNOWN TO BE HARMFUL

Antihistamines	Ethamsylate	Quinidine
Cimetidine	Ethosuximide	Ranitidine
Diltiazem	Minoxidil	Spironolactone
Erythromycin	Pyrimethamine	Trimethoprim

DRUGS KNOWN TO BE PRESENT IN MILK IN AMOUNTS THAT ARE PROBABLY TOO SMALL TO BE HARMFUL AT USUAL THERAPEUTIC DOSES

Acetazolamide	Fenoprofen	Nitrazepam
ACTH	Flecainide	Nizatidine
Azathioprine	Flupenthixol	Paracetamol
Baclofen	Flurbiprofen	Phenylbutazone
Buprenorphine	Fluvoxamine	Phenytoin
Captopril	Frusemide	Pirenzepine
Carbamazepine	Haloperidol	Piroxicam
Chlormethiazole	Heparin	Procainamide
Chloroquine	Hydralazine	Pyrazinamide
Chlorprothixene	Hydroxychloroquine	Pyridostigmine
Cisapride	Hyoscine	Rifampicin
Clavulanic acid	Ibuprofen	Sodium valproate
(Augmentin)	Insulin	Terbutaline
Codeine	Ketoprofen	Thiazide diuretics
Cycloserine	Loprazolam	Tiaprofenic acid
Dextropropoxyphene	Mebeverine	Tolmetin
Diclofenac	Mefenamic acid	Trazodone
Digoxin	Methyldopa	Tricyclic
Disopyramide	Metoclopramide	antidepressants
Domperidone	Mexiletine	Verapamil
Enalapril	Mianserin	Warfarin
Ethambutol	Naproxen	Zopiclone
Famotidine	Nefopam	Zuclopenthixol
Fenbufen	Nifedipine	

Index